HERBAL REMEDIES FOR BUSY WOMEN

57 HARD HITTING HERBS TO EFFECTIVELY TARGET MENOPAUSE, STRESS, GUT HEALTH AND OTHER COMMON AILMENTS AS PART OF YOUR NORMAL DAILY ROUTINE

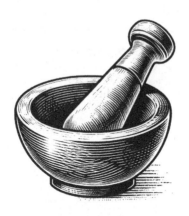

CONTENTS

3

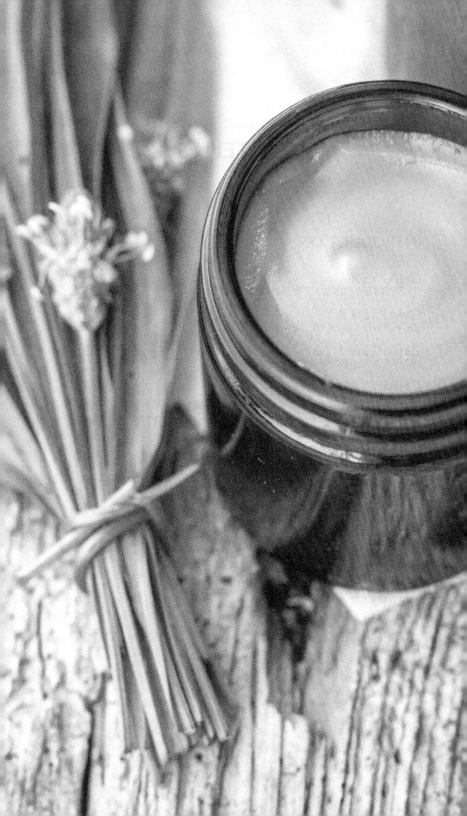

INTRODUCTION

In today's fast-paced world, finding a moment for oneself, let alone for one's health, can feel like an insurmountable challenge, especially for women juggling multiple roles. Yet, what if I told you there is a way to integrate natural healing into your hectic schedule that is both simple and effective? This book is a testament to the power of herbal remedies, tailored specifically to cater to the needs of busy women seeking to enhance their health naturally and lessen their reliance on prescription and over-the-counter medication in support of day to day living.

This book aims to simplify the often, complex world of herbal medicine for you. Whether you are a novice curious about herbal teas or a busy mom seeking natural salves for your family, the practical steps provided here will guide you to create your own herbal remedies with ease. From soothing tinctures to healing poultices, you'll learn how to craft these in your own home, integrating health and wellness seamlessly into your daily life. Safety and efficacy are paramount. Detailed discussions on the potential side effects, interactions with medications, and specific health conditions are included to ensure you use herbal remedies safely. All herbs profiled in this book come with health benefits, practical uses, and safety considerations, making them a reliable resource for your herbal remedy needs.

Moreover, this book is enriched with historical anecdotes, points of cultural significance and summaries of scientific studies, that not only provide a deeper understanding of the herbs, but also strengthen your trust in their efficacy. I recognize some readers may be skeptical about turning to leaves and roots for health benefits. It is natural to question new approaches, especially in an age dominated by modern medicine. I address these concerns with clear, evidence-based information that respects both traditional wisdom and contemporary scientific insights.

I invite you to join me on this transformative journey into the world of herbal remedies. Let this be your gateway to discovering the profound impact these plants can have on your health and well-being. Together, let's embrace the natural path to healing, one leaf at a time.

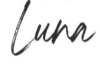

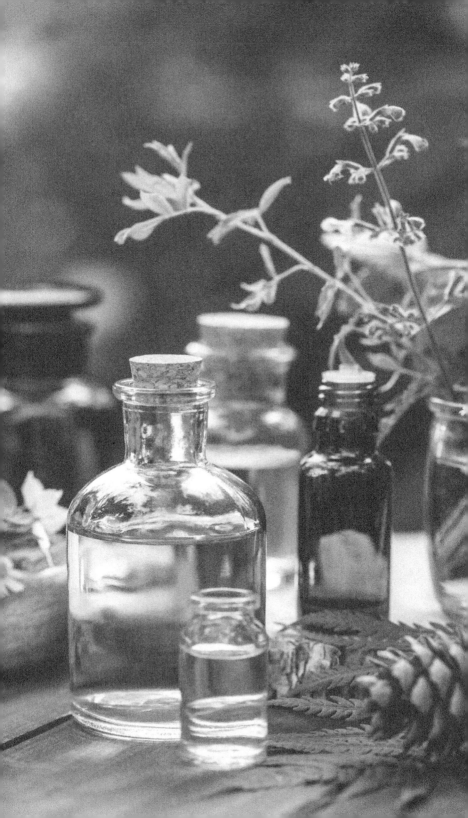

CHAPTER I
UNDERSTANDING HERBAL REMEDIES

In a world bustling with quick fixes and fast-paced solutions, the ancient wisdom of herbal remedies offers a refreshing, grounded approach to personal health and wellness. Often, the simplest changes to our daily routines can prompt the most profound improvements in our overall well-being. This chapter opens the door to the foundational knowledge of herbal medicine, designed specifically with you in mind - a vibrant woman steering through the demands of modern life. As we explore the richness of herbal remedies, you will discover not only how to use these natural wonders but also understand the language and forms they come in, which are as varied and rich as the cultures from which they stem.

1.1 Herbal Medicine: Terminology Simplified

To fully appreciate and effectively utilize herbal remedies, it's crucial to begin with a clear grasp of the key terms used in herbal medicine. Terms like 'tincture,' 'infusion,' 'decoction,' and 'poultice' frequently appear in texts and discussions related to herbal treatments. Each term denotes a specific type of herbal preparation. An 'infusion' is what you might know as herbal tea, typically made by steeping leaves or flowers in hot water. A 'decoction' involves simmering tougher plant materials like roots or bark to extract their vital constituents. Understanding these terms is not just about expanding your vocabulary, it's about deepening your relationship with herbal medicine, enabling you to follow recipes and make effective use of herbal remedies.

Herbal medicine comes in various forms, each suitable for different types of applications and treatments. Tinctures are concentrated herbal extracts made by soaking herbs in alcohol or vinegar, a method that extracts a broader spectrum of plant constituents than water alone can. Salves and balms are semi-solid preparations used for external application, often made from oils and waxes infused with herbs to treat skin issues or deliver other healing compounds directly through the skin. Poultices involve fresh or dried herbs applied directly to the skin, sometimes wrapped or bandaged, to provide relief for inflammation, pain, or to draw out infections.

Application Methods

The method of applying or consuming an herbal remedy can significantly affect its efficiency and appropriateness for certain conditions. Teas and infusions are generally ingested and can be excellent for their calming, systemic effects or for treating internal ailments. Tinctures, being more concentrated, are taken in small quantities and are beneficial for long-term treatment of conditions like chronic pain or anxiety. Topically applied forms such as salves and poultices provide targeted relief and are ideal for localized issues such as wounds, bruises, or arthritis. Each application method leverages the unique properties of herbs in a form that best suits the healing need.

The Language of Herbs

Herbalism is as much about the science of plants as it is about their lore and history. Phrases such as 'adaptogen' or 'alterative' are not just fancy terms but categories that help us understand how herbs act within the body. Adaptogens, for example, help the body adapt to stress and exert a normalizing effect upon bodily processes. Alteratives are known as 'blood purifiers' and influence the body's detoxification pathways. Learning this language does more than aid in comprehension; it connects you to centuries of herbalist tradition - a continuum of healing wisdom passed through generations.

Understanding the intricacies of using herbal remedies empowers you, not only to make informed choices about your health, but also to engage with a community of global tradition that supports natural and holistic living.

As you become more familiar with the terminology and applications, you'll find that incorporating herbal medicine into your life becomes an act of self-care that harmonizes body, mind, and spirit.

1.2 Safety First: Side Effects and Interactions

When weaving the vibrant threads of herbal remedies into the fabric of your daily life, it becomes imperative to address the safety aspects with the same enthusiasm as their benefits. Natural does not always mean safe for everyone, and understanding this distinction is crucial. Every herb comes with its own set of characteristics, and while many are gentle and beneficial, others can pose potential risks if not used correctly. It is vital to educate yourself on how to identify and understand the possible risks associated with certain herbs. For instance, while chamomile is widely regarded for its calming effects, it can cause allergic reactions in individuals sensitive to the Asteraceae family, which includes ragweed and chrysanthemums. Recognizing signs of an allergic reaction, which could range from skin rashes to respiratory issues, is a fundamental skill for anyone using herbal remedies.

Interactions between herbal preparations and pharmaceutical medications form another critical area of focus. Many herbs can alter the effectiveness of drugs, either diminishing their therapeutic effect or exacerbating their side effects. St. John's Wort, celebrated for its ability to alleviate depression, may lead to increased sensitivity to sunlight, which many might not anticipate, but can also interfere with the effectiveness of birth control pills and other medications. Therefore, it is essential to consult healthcare providers about potential interactions if you are taking prescribed medications. This practice ensures that your holistic and conventional treatments complement rather than contradict each other.

Listening to your body serves as an invaluable guide in using herbal remedies safely. The body often sends signals when something is amiss, and tuning into these cues can prevent the escalation of adverse reactions. For example, if you notice unusual fatigue or digestive discomfort after starting a new herbal tea, it could be your body's way of signaling intolerance or a negative reaction to the herb. It is important to start with small doses and observe how your body responds during the initial days. This cautious approach not only helps in identifying adverse reactions early but also allows you to adjust dosages or discontinue use under safer conditions.

Knowing when to seek advice from a healthcare professional is a crucial judgment call that can safeguard your health. While herbal remedies can be excellent for managing minor ailments and enhancing overall wellness, they are not substitutes for professional medical treatment in the face of serious health issues. If symptoms persist or worsen, or if you suspect that an herb might be contributing to health issues, it is imperative to consult a medical professional. This is particularly important for persistent issues such as prolonged digestive problems, severe allergic reactions, or any symptoms that interfere with daily activities. Medical professionals can provide comprehensive assessments that consider both your conventional and herbal treatment options, ensuring a holistic approach to your health that is both safe and effective.

1.3 The Herbal Pantry: Herbs for Women's Health

In cultivating a harmonious lifestyle, the creation of a personalized herbal pantry becomes a pivotal step. This specially curated collection not only nurtures your body but also supports your mind and spirit, particularly addressing the unique health challenges women often face. The herbs chosen for your pantry should reflect not only their health benefits but also your personal health goals and needs. For instance, herbs like ginger and turmeric are renowned not only for their culinary uses but also for their potent anti-inflammatory properties, making them indispensable in a woman's herbal arsenal for managing everything from menstrual cramps to arthritis. Lavender and chamomile are staples for their soothing and calming effects, ideal for stress relief and promoting a restful sleep. For those dealing with hormonal imbalances, chaste tree berry (Vitex) and maca root are invaluable for regulating hormonal functions and supporting reproductive health.

Building your herbal collection begins with understanding the versatility and efficacy of each herb. A well-stocked pantry should include a diverse range of herbs to allow for a comprehensive approach to health. Start with versatile herbs that can be used in multiple ways. For example, nettle is a powerhouse of nutrients, known for its ability to support iron levels in the body, making it particularly beneficial during menstruation or pregnancy. It can be used as a tea, added to soups, or even included in smoothies. Similarly, dandelion, often overlooked as a common weed, is a fantastic liver cleanser and can be used both as a digestive aid and a skin detoxifier. When selecting herbs, consider those that can be easily integrated into your daily diet or routine, thereby enhancing their practical use and benefits.

Addressing specific women's health issues through targeted herbal remedies allows for proactive management of your health. Hormonal balance, for instance, can be supported by incorporating ashwagandha, which acts as an adaptogen to help the body manage stress, a common disruptor of hormonal equilibrium. Red raspberry leaf is highly praised for its uterine toning properties, making it a valuable herb during pregnancy and for menstrual health. For those seeking natural remedies for menopausal symptoms, black cohosh offers a significant reduction in hot flashes and mood swings. It's about choosing herbs that not only address specific symptoms but also contribute to overall well-being.

Sustainability in sourcing herbs is not just an ethical commitment but a quality assurance measure that impacts the efficacy of your herbal remedies. Opting for ethically sourced herbs ensures that the products are grown without harmful pesticides and harvested in a manner that supports the environment and the communities involved in their cultivation. This practice not only contributes to the health of the planet but also ensures that you are receiving the highest quality product. When possible, purchase herbs from local growers or organic suppliers who can provide detailed information about their farming and harvesting practices. This transparency allows you to make informed choices that align with your health and environmental values.

In creating your herbal pantry, consider not only the health benefits and uses of each herb but also the broader impact of your choices on personal and environmental health. By choosing sustainably sourced, versatile herbs that address specific women's health issues, you are investing in a holistic approach to wellness that nurtures both the body and the environment. This thoughtful selection and use of herbs empower you to take control of your health in a way that is reflective of your values and needs, paving the way for a healthier, more balanced life.

1.4 Quality Matters: Sourcing and Storing Your Herbs

Navigating the realm of herbal remedies requires more than just knowledge of their uses; understanding where your herbs come from and how they are kept can drastically affect their healing properties. The journey from soil to shelf is fraught with factors that can either preserve the vitality of these botanicals or diminish it. As someone deeply rooted in the holistic wellness community, I've come to realize that the quality of the herbs we use is as crucial as the remedies themselves. Here, I will guide you through finding reputable sources and distinguishing between organic and non-organic choices, ensuring that the herbs you select bring the utmost benefit to your health.

The quest for high-quality herbs begins with choosing the right suppliers. In an ideal world, we would all have access to an herbal garden, but for many, this isn't practical. Thus, finding trustworthy vendors becomes essential. Start by seeking out local apothecaries or health food stores with knowledgeable staff who can provide detailed information about their herb sources.

These establishments often maintain rigorous standards for the products they stock. Additionally, attending herbal conferences or workshops not only deepens your understanding but also connects you with seasoned herbalists who can recommend reliable suppliers. A good resource to begin your research is the AHPA (American Herbal Products Association).

For those who prefer the convenience of online shopping, it's vital to vet internet retailers thoroughly. Look for suppliers who provide extensive details about their herbs, including where they are grown, their harvesting methods, and any testing they undergo for purity and potency. Websites that feature customer reviews can offer insights into the quality of herbs and the reliability of the vendor. Furthermore, reputable online suppliers often provide certificates of analysis for their herbs, which are conducted by third-party labs and offer proof of their quality and safety.

Reputable online suppliers that you might like to try:

www.starwest-botanicals.com
www.mountainroseherbs.com
www.thegrowers-exchange.com

The debate between using organic and non-organic herbs is not just about personal health; it encompasses environmental ethics and practices as well. Organic herbs are grown without synthetic pesticides, herbicides, or fertilizers, all of which can leave residues on plants that not only compromise your health but also harm the ecosystem. The organic cultivation process supports biodiversity, conserves water, and enhances the soil's health, which in turn supports the plants' nutritional and medicinal qualities. When you choose organic, you are not only investing in your health but also contributing to sustainable agricultural practices that respect our planet.

However, it's important to recognize that some small-scale farmers who follow organic farming methods may not have official organic certification due to the cost and complexity of the certification process. In these cases, building a relationship with your herb supplier can help you learn about their farming practices and make informed choices, even if their herbs are not officially certified.

Once you have sourced your high-quality herbs, proper storage is key to preserving their medicinal properties. Light, heat, and moisture are the main enemies of dried herbs. They can degrade active compounds and encourage the growth of mold and bacteria. To avoid this, store herbs in airtight containers made of materials that do not react with contents, such as glass or stainless steel. Place these containers in a cool, dark place like a cupboard or a pantry to protect them from light and heat. If properly stored, most dried herbs can retain their potency for up to one year, though some, like flowers and leaves, are best used within six months for maximum efficacy. For those who use fresh herbs, remember that these require different handling. Fresh herbs can be kept in the refrigerator, generally wrapped in a damp cloth or paper towel and sealed in a reusable bag to maintain moisture without becoming soggy. Some herbs, like basil, prefer to be kept at room temperature with their stems in water. Always check for any signs of wilting or mold, which indicate that the herb's quality is declining.

Being able to identify high-quality herbs by appearance, smell, and texture is crucial. Good quality dried herbs should retain vibrant colors, indicative of strong active constituents and proper drying and storage methods. They should smell fresh and aromatic, a key indicator of their potency. If an herb smells musty or has no scent, it's likely lost its medicinal properties. The texture should also be considered; leaves and flowers should crumble under slight pressure, not turn to dust or feel leathery, both of which suggest improper drying.

For fresh herbs, look for perky, vibrant leaves without any brown spots or signs of wilting. Fresh herbs should feel firm and spring back when gently pressed, not feel limp or dry. By educating yourself on these quality indicators, you empower yourself to make the best choices for your herbal treatments, ensuring that you derive the maximum benefit from each remedy you prepare.

1.5 Tailoring Herbal Remedies to Your Body's Needs

Personalizing your approach to herbal remedies is not just a practice; it's a transformation that aligns your health regimen with your individual needs and life phases. Each woman's body communicates differently and also reacts uniquely to herbal treatments, which means that the effectiveness of a herb can vary widely from one individual to another. This variability underscores the importance of customizing herbal remedies to fit personal health conditions and lifestyles. For instance, while chamomile might work wonders for one person's sleep issues, another might find lavender more effective. Starting with understanding your specific health goals - be it improving sleep, reducing anxiety, or managing menstrual pain - allows you to select herbs that are most likely to benefit your particular conditions.

When personalizing herbal treatments, consider not only the desired health benefits but also any existing health conditions or allergies. For example, if you have a thyroid condition, herbs like lemon balm or ashwagandha might be particularly beneficial. However, it's crucial to adjust dosages and combinations to see what works best for you, keeping in mind that less is often more when beginning a new herbal regimen. Gradually increasing the dosage can help your body adapt without overwhelming it, allowing you to monitor the effects and make adjustments as needed. This method helps in identifying the optimal mix and amount that provides relief without adverse effects.

Understanding your body's signals plays a crucial role in effectively personalizing and adjusting your herbal treatments. Just as a gardener learns to read the signs of their plants' needs, you too can learn to interpret your body's responses to different herbs. Paying close attention to how you feel after taking a herb - whether you notice improvement in your symptoms, experience side effects, or see no change at all - is key. This might mean noticing whether your sleep improves with valerian root or if ginger tea helps reduce your digestive discomfort. It's important to observe both the subtle and significant changes in your symptoms and overall well-being.

Keeping a wellness journal can be an invaluable tool in this process. Documenting which herbs you take, the amounts, the time of day, and the effects you notice, can help you track patterns and outcomes more clearly. This documentation provides insights that are critical in refining your herbal strategy. Over time, this journal will become a personalized health ledger, offering a clear view of what works, what doesn't, and how your body's needs may change over time.

As women, we navigate numerous physiological changes through different stages of life - from menstrual cycles to pregnancy, to menopause. Each stage has unique health requirements and challenges, and herbal remedies can be adapted to meet these changing needs. During reproductive years, herbs like raspberry leaf can support uterine health, while during menopause, sage might be introduced to help reduce hot flashes. The key is to remain attuned to the body's shifting needs and to adjust your herbal practices accordingly. For younger women, the focus might be on herbs that help with menstrual regularity and fertility, while older women might prioritize herbs that support bone health and hormonal balance.

Adjusting your herbal remedies as you transition through life stages not only helps in managing the specific health challenges of each phase but also supports optimal health throughout your life. With each change, whether it's adjusting dosages or introducing new herbs into your regimen, you reaffirm your commitment to nurturing your body. This adaptive, responsive approach ensures that your herbal treatment strategy remains effective, relevant, and tailored to your body's evolving needs.

1.6 Adding Herbs Seamlessly into Your Daily Routine

Integrating herbal remedies into your daily life need not be a daunting overhaul of your current lifestyle; rather, it can be a graceful and enriching enhancement. Starting small is key to making this integration feel less like a chore and more like a naturally evolving part of your everyday routine. Consider beginning with a single herb that addresses a specific need, such as chamomile for better sleep or ginger for digestion. You might start by introducing a nightly cup of chamomile tea before bed or adding fresh ginger to your morning smoothie. These small steps help to familiarize you with the herb's effects and flavors, making the experience both manageable and enjoyable.

As you grow more comfortable and knowledgeable, gradually expand your repertoire. Incorporating herbal remedies can be as simple as adding a spoonful of cinnamon to your oatmeal to help stabilize blood sugar levels or tossing a handful of fresh basil into your pasta for its anti-inflammatory benefits. The key is to weave these practices into your existing habits rather than creating entirely new routines that might feel a little overwhelming. Over time, these small incorporations will form a tapestry of wellness that naturally fits into the rhythm of your day-to-day life.

The choice between using herbal supplements and whole herbs is significant and worth considering. Supplements, often available in capsules, tinctures, or powders, offer convenience and precise dosing, which can be particularly beneficial for those with hectic schedules. They are a straightforward way to ensure you are getting specific amounts of active herbal constituents and can be especially useful when targeting specific health issues. However, it's crucial to source high-quality supplements from reputable suppliers to avoid contaminants and ensure potency.

On the other hand, using whole herbs - whether fresh or dried - provides a sensory experience that can deepen your connection to the remedies you are using. Preparing a meal or a cup of tea with whole herbs allows you to engage with the colors, textures, and aromas of the plants, enriching the healing process. Furthermore, whole herbs typically offer a broader range of health-supporting constituents than what might be present in an extract or capsule. They also allow for greater flexibility in how you use them, encouraging creativity in your culinary and wellness practices.

Finding creative ways to incorporate herbs into your daily routine can transform what might seem like a mundane task into a delightful ritual. Herbs can be infused in waters, blended into smoothies, brewed into teas, or even added to bathwater for a relaxing soak. Consider starting your day with a refreshing glass of water infused with cucumber and mint to stimulate digestion and hydrate your body. Or perhaps unwind after a long day with a soothing bath steeped with lavender and chamomile, which not only calms the mind but also benefits the skin.

Herbal-infused oils can be used in cooking or as salad dressings, adding both flavor and health benefits to your meals. For instance, rosemary-infused olive oil not only elevates the taste of roasted vegetables but also incorporates rosemary's memory-boosting properties into your diet. Similarly, incorporating herbal vinegars, such as those infused with dandelion or garlic, into your cooking can enhance both the nutritional profile and the flavor complexity of your dishes.

Building an herbal habit that lasts involves setting realistic goals and being patient with yourself as you learn and grow in your herbal practices. Consistency is more critical than intensity; a small daily action is more beneficial than an occasional grand gesture. To make this practice stick, tie your new herbal habits to existing routines. For example, if you already have a habit of drinking a morning cup of coffee, consider switching to an herbal coffee substitute like chicory root from time to time, which can offer liver support and reduce caffeine intake.

Alternatively, if you enjoy reading in the evening, create a ritual of sipping a calming herbal tea while you do so.

Additionally, keeping your herbs visible and easily accessible can remind you to use them regularly. Store your teas and dried herbs near your cooking area or keep a small herb garden on a windowsill where you'll see it every day. Visibility not only reminds you to use your herbs but also keeps the beauty and natural diversity of these plants at the forefront of your mind, enhancing your daily life not just physically but also spiritually and aesthetically. Ultimately, the goal is to make herbal practices a seamless, enjoyable part of your daily life, nurturing your body and enriching your routines with natural, health-supporting habits. As these practices become ingrained, they will feel less like tasks and more like cherished parts of your daily rhythm, contributing to a holistic sense of wellbeing that supports you through every aspect of your busy life.

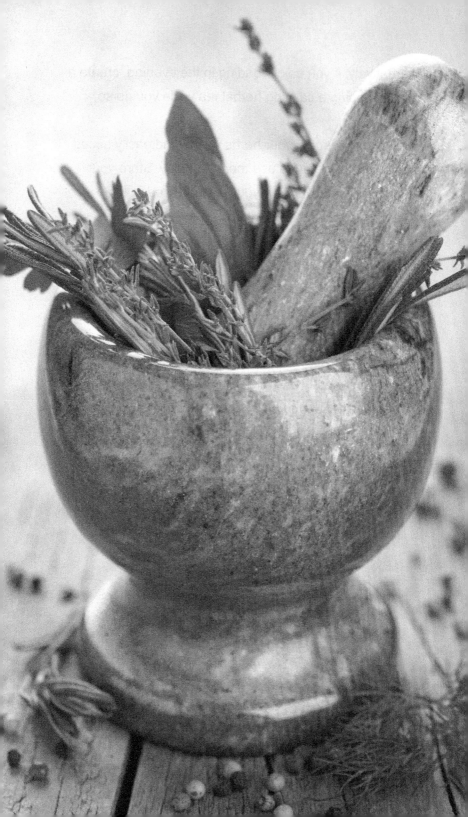

CHAPTER 2
CRAFTING YOUR HERBAL REMEDIES

In the enchanting world of herbal medicine, the profound art of crafting your own remedies opens a new dimension of personal empowerment and connection to the natural world. Imagine harnessing the curative powers of plants and herbs, transforming them into potent remedies that resonate with your body's unique rhythms and needs. Tinctures, with their concentrated essence, offer a convenient and effective way to utilize the therapeutic properties of herbs. Whether you are looking to soothe a restless mind, alleviate chronic discomfort, or bolster your immune system, tinctures can be a remarkable addition to your wellness toolkit. Let's embark on this detailed exploration of making tinctures, ensuring you feel confident and equipped to begin this rewarding practice.

2.1 Making Tinctures: A Step-by-Step Guide

Tinctures are alcohol-based extracts that capture the active compounds of herbs, preserving their medicinal qualities for extended periods. The process of making tinctures is both an art and a science, accessible to beginners yet refined enough for seasoned herbalists. To start, you will need a few basic tools: a clean glass jar with a tight-fitting lid, high-proof alcohol (such as vodka or brandy), your herb of choice, a strainer, and dark glass bottles for storage. The beauty of tincture making lies in its simplicity and the profound connection it fosters with the healing plants.

The choice of solvent is crucial in tincture making. While high-proof alcohol is a popular choice due to its efficiency in extracting a wide range of plant constituents and its preservative properties, other solvents like glycerin or vinegar can also be used, particularly for those who prefer to avoid alcohol. Alcohol, with at least 40% alcohol content, is most effective at preserving the tincture and extracting both water-soluble and alcohol-soluble compounds, making it a versatile choice for most herbs. Glycerin, a sweet-tasting solvent, is suitable for creating alcohol-free tinctures, ideal for children or those sensitive to alcohol, though it may not extract as wide a range of compounds. Vinegar, rich in acetic acid, offers health benefits of its own and is a good choice for extracting minerals from herbs.

Creating your first tincture involves a few straightforward steps:

1. **Select and Prepare Your Herb**: Choose fresh or dried herbs. Fresh herbs should be free from pesticides and not wilted, while dried herbs should be aromatic and not too crumbly.
2. **Chop or Grind the Herbs**: This increases the surface area and facilitates a more thorough extraction.
3. **Fill the Jar**: Place the herbs in your glass jar, filling it halfway for fresh herbs, or one-quarter for dried herbs, as dried herbs expand when soaked.
4. **Add the Solvent**: Pour the alcohol over the herbs until the jar is nearly full. Ensure that the herbs are completely submerged to prevent mold growth.
5. **Seal and Store**: Close the jar tightly and store it in a cool, dark place. Shake the jar daily for the first week to mix the contents and aid in the extraction process.
6. **Strain and Bottle**: After 4-6 weeks, strain the tincture through a fine mesh strainer or cheese cloth into dark glass bottles. Label the bottles with the herb and date of production.

Proper storage is key to maintaining the potency of your tinctures. Store them in a cabinet or a pantry or another easily accessible cool, dark place, away from direct sunlight. When stored correctly, tinctures can last several years. To use the tincture, a standard dose is typically 1-2 ml, taken 1-3 times daily. However, dosages can vary based on the herb and the individual's needs, so it's important to do some research or consult with a healthcare provider. Tinctures can be taken directly under the tongue for fast absorption or added to a small amount of water or tea. Integrating tinctures into your daily routine can enhance your wellness in powerful ways. For instance, a tincture made from ginger can be taken with meals to aid digestion or at the first sign of nausea. A chamomile tincture might be used in the evening to promote relaxation and support healthy sleep patterns. For those managing chronic conditions, such as arthritis, a turmeric tincture could be a valuable anti-inflammatory addition to their daily regimen.

Crafting your own tinctures not only empowers you to take control of your health care, it also deepens your connection to the natural world, providing a tangible link between the healing power of plants and your personal wellness journey. With each drop, these potent extracts bring the ancient wisdom of herbal medicine into your everyday life, offering a profound reminder of nature's capacity to nourish and heal.

2.2 Teas for Every Mood: Blending Techniques

The creation of herbal teas is a delightful craft that combines the pleasures of taste and the benefits of medicinal properties, all steeped into a warm, comforting cup. In this exploration of herbal tea blending, you'll discover how to harmonize flavors while targeting specific wellness needs, making each sip a purposeful step towards better health. The art of blending herbal teas involves more than just mixing a few herbs together; it requires an understanding of the individual properties of each herb, how they interact with each other, and the effects they have on the body and mind.

When beginning your tea blending journey, consider first the purpose of the tea. Are you aiming to calm a busy mind, soothe a troublesome stomach, or perhaps invigorate your morning routine? Each goal might lead you towards different herbs. For instance, a tea blended for sleep may feature chamomile and lavender, known for their soothing and relaxing properties, while a digestive aid might lean on peppermint and ginger to ease stomach discomfort. Once the purpose is clear, think about the flavor profiles of these herbs and how they might complement or contrast each other to create a pleasing blend.

Balancing taste and potency is crucial; some herbs have strong flavors that can overpower others, while some

33

have subtle notes that might be lost in a blend. For example, the robust flavor of hibiscus can dominate a tea blend, so it should be used sparingly unless it's the intended dominant note. Similarly, delicate herbs like lemon balm might need to be used in greater quantities or combined with other mild herbs to maintain their presence in the blend. The key is to start with small amounts, gradually adjusting your recipe until you find the perfect balance that meets both your flavor preferences and wellness goals.

Herbal teas can be wonderfully effective for managing everyday ailments, and crafting your own blends allows you to tailor them to your specific needs. For stress relief, a blend of chamomile, lavender, and lemon balm can work wonders. Chamomile is not only soothing but also mildly sedative, while lavender helps reduce anxiety, and lemon balm boosts mood. To prepare, use one part chamomile, one part lavender, and two parts lemon balm. Steep in hot water for 5 to 10 minutes for a calming evening drink.

For those nights when sleep seems elusive, try a blend of valerian root, passionflower, and hops. Valerian root is a powerful herbal sedative, passionflower helps to quiet the mind, and hops add a pleasantly bitter flavor while enhancing the blend's sedative properties. Mix one part valerian root, one part passionflower, and one part hops.

Since valerian root is quite potent, it's wise to start with a small dose to see how you respond before adjusting the blend.

Digestive discomfort can be alleviated with a simple tea made from peppermint, ginger, and fennel. Peppermint soothes the stomach, ginger aids digestion and reduces nausea, and fennel helps to relieve gas and bloating. Combine two parts peppermint, one part ginger, and one part fennel. This tea is not only effective but also has a refreshing and invigorating taste, making it perfect after meals.

The technique of brewing herbal tea is as important as the blend itself. To maximize the medicinal benefits, cover your teapot or cup while steeping to prevent the escape of aromatic compounds and steam, which contain therapeutic essential oils. Most herbal teas benefit from a longer steeping time than traditional teas; allowing them to steep for 10 to 15 minutes will generally result in a stronger, more beneficial tea. Water temperature is also crucial and varies depending on the herbs used. Delicate herbs like chamomile and lavender are best steeped in water that's just below boiling, to preserve their delicate oils and flavors. In contrast, tougher, more fibrous herbs like ginger and valerian root can handle boiling water, which helps to extract their full range of medicinal compounds.

Presenting and storing your herbal teas should be both practical and pleasing. For daily ease, store your blends in clear, airtight containers, keeping them in your pantry to preserve their flavors and medicinal properties. When serving, consider the visual appeal and the sensory experience. Use transparent teapots or cups to showcase the beauty of the herbal blend, and perhaps add a garnish that complements the tea's ingredients, like a sprig of mint or a slice of lemon.

For those special moments, or when sharing your blends with others, the presentation can elevate the experience. Serve tea in fine china or artisan-crafted pottery to celebrate the art of herbal tea making or, for a more modern take, consider a glass tea set. If you prefer this more modern aesthetic, use mineral water to make the tea for a purer, more superior taste and to lessen the likelihood of a petrol-like film forming on the surface of the tea - this is usually present when oils in the tea react with impurities in the water. Each element, from the container to the cup, adds a layer of enjoyment, making each sip a more profound acknowledgment of the healing powers of nature.

Each of these elements - from the choice and balance of herbs to the brewing and presentation - contributes to the transformation of simple ingredients into a healing, enjoyable beverage. Through this process, you not only create a tea that benefits the body but also cultivate a deeper appreciation and connection to the natural world, enhancing your overall wellness journey.

2.3 Soothing Salves: Natural Solutions for Skin Care

The allure of herbal salves lies in their simplicity and the profound soothing they offer to the skin, making them a cherished component in natural skincare routines. A salve is essentially a healing balm made from oils infused with herbs, thickened with beeswax to create a semi-solid state. This form allows for the herbs' medicinal properties to be absorbed directly through the skin, providing targeted relief and nourishment. Herbal salves can be especially beneficial for addressing a variety of skin conditions such as dryness, irritation, and minor wounds, or simply for enhancing skin health and resilience.

Creating your own herbal salves at home not only allows you to customize ingredients to suit your specific skin needs but also ensures that you are using the freshest, most natural products. Here's a detailed guide to making your first herbal salve: Begin by selecting your herbs. For healing and soothing properties, calendula and chamomile are excellent choices due to their anti-inflammatory and gentle healing effects. If you're aiming for a more antiseptic salve, herbs like lavender and tea tree offer potent antimicrobial benefits. Once you've chosen your herbs, the next step is to infuse them into a carrier oil. Olive oil is a popular choice for its antioxidant properties, but almond oil can be a lighter alternative that also nourishes the skin.

Place the herbs in a jar and cover them with oil so they are fully submerged. Seal the jar and place it in a warm, sunny spot to infuse for about two weeks, or gently heat the oil and herbs in a double boiler for a few hours if you're short on time. Once the oil is infused, strain out the herbs with cheesecloth, ensuring all plant matter is removed. The final step is to gently heat the infused oil and mix it with beeswax until the wax is fully melted. Pour the mixture into clean containers and allow it to cool and set. The result is a beautiful, natural salve that's ready for use.

Herbal salves can be applied directly to the skin on areas that need healing or moisturizing. Apply a small amount to cuts, scrapes, rashes, or just dry skin areas. The salve works by creating a protective barrier on the skin that also delivers the healing properties of the herbs deep into the skin layers.

Key Ingredients for Effective Salves

When crafting salves, the selection of carrier oils and essential oils alongside the primary herbs can significantly influence the effectiveness and sensory qualities of your final product. Carrier oils serve as the base in which your chosen herbs are infused and play a crucial role in the texture and therapeutic properties of the salve. Coconut oil, for example, is rich in fatty acids that are excellent for moisturizing and healing damaged skin. Jojoba oil, while technically a wax, mimics the skin's natural sebum, making it particularly effective for facial applications without clogging pores.

To enhance the medicinal power of your salve, consider incorporating essential oils. These highly concentrated plant extracts add not only therapeutic benefits but also pleasant aromas. For a calming salve, adding a few drops of lavender essential oil can enhance the relaxing effects, making it perfect for use before sleep. For a more invigorating salve, peppermint essential oil can stimulate circulation and soothe tired, aching muscles. However, it's important to use essential oils sparingly and cautiously, as their high concentration can be irritating to the skin if overused. Typically, a few drops per ounce of carrier oil are sufficient.

Application and Storage

Applying herbal salves effectively is key to maximizing their healing benefits. Always start with clean, dry skin to prevent trapping any bacteria under the salve. Scoop a small amount onto your fingers and gently massage it into the skin until it's absorbed. The warmth of your skin will soften the salve, making it easier to spread. It's particularly effective when applied to damp skin, such as after a shower, as this helps lock in moisture. Storing your salves correctly ensures they maintain their potency and prevent spoilage. Since natural salves don't contain preservatives, as with any herbal mixture, they are best kept in a cool, dark place to extend their shelf life. Small tins or glass jars with tight-fitting lids are ideal containers as they prevent exposure to air and light, both of which can degrade the salve over time. If stored properly, most herbal salves can last for up to a year. Always check for any changes in smell, texture, or color, which can indicate that the salve is past its best and should be replaced.

Creating and using your own herbal salves is not only a deeply satisfying way to engage with the natural world but also an effective approach to skin care that puts you in control of the ingredients you apply to your body. As you explore different herbs, oils, and blends, you'll likely find that these salves become an indispensable part of your wellness routine, offering a tangible connection to the healing power of nature.

2.4 Crafting Poultices for Pain Relief and Healing

Poultices represent one of the most traditional forms of herbal remedies, offering direct, potent healing benefits especially when it comes to localized pain and inflammation. Essentially, a poultice involves the use of fresh or dried herbs and other therapeutic substances that are applied directly to the skin, where their healing properties can penetrate the underlying tissues. The moisture content of the poultice, combined with the natural medicinal qualities of the herbs, can provide significant relief for a variety of ailments, including bruises, infections, aches, and skin irritations.

Understanding when and how to use a poultice can significantly enhance its effectiveness. Poultices are particularly beneficial for treating localized swelling, muscle pains, boils, and abscesses. They work by increasing blood flow to the affected area, reducing inflammation, and accelerating healing. The warmth or coolness of a poultice, depending on its preparation, also plays a crucial role in its healing properties. Warm poultices are excellent for soothing sore muscles or relieving tightness, while cool poultices can help reduce swelling and calm inflamed skin. Creating your first poultice is straightforward and involves a few simple steps. Begin by selecting an appropriate herb based on the condition you wish to treat. For instance, crushed fresh ginger is excellent for inflammatory conditions and pain, whereas calendula works well for skin healing and mild infections. Once you've chosen your herb, you need to form a paste. This can be done by grinding the herb with a mortar and pestle, adding a small amount of warm water or oil to reach the desired consistency. If you're using dried herbs, they may need to be moistened and heated slightly to activate their therapeutic properties. Spread this paste directly onto the skin or onto a soft cloth if the skin is broken or highly sensitive, then apply it to the affected area.

For conditions such as sprains or arthritis, where deeper tissue penetration is needed, you can enhance the poultice's effectiveness by layering it with plastic wrap and a warm cloth. This method helps maintain the poultice's moisture and warmth, increasing the absorption of the herbal constituents. Secure the poultice with a bandage or wrap to keep it in place, but ensure it's not so tight that it cuts off circulation.

Herbs to Use for Different Conditions

The choice of herbs is critical in crafting an effective poultice. Each herb has specific properties that make it particularly beneficial for certain conditions. For skin infections and minor wounds, turmeric is highly recommended due to its powerful antibacterial and anti-inflammatory properties. For bruises and sprains, arnica is beneficial, but it should be used with caution as it is not suitable for broken skin. Comfrey, known as 'knitbone', is excellent for broken bones and sprains for its ability to promote rapid healing. However, it should not be used on open wounds due to its rapid healing properties that can lead to tissue forming over an unhealed infection. It is also important to stress that the use of comfrey for broken bones is not a substitute for professional medical attention, more a supplemental treatment.

When dealing with eczema or skin rashes, an oatmeal poultice can be soothing and healing. Oatmeal is not only gentle on the skin but also possesses anti-inflammatory properties that help calm the irritation and itchiness associated with these conditions. For a more cooling effect, particularly for conditions like sunburn or reactive skin flare-ups, aloe vera combined with cucumber in a poultice provides immediate cooling relief and promotes healing.

Applying and Removing Poultices

Applying a poultice correctly is as important as making one. Ensure the area of application is clean before applying the poultice to prevent any potential infection. Spread the herb paste thickly over the area, covering it with a clean cloth if not applied directly to the skin. For an inflamed or painful area, you might want to secure the poultice with a wrap but make sure it's loose enough to allow blood flow. The duration for which a poultice should be left in place can vary, but generally, it's between 1 to

24 hours, depending on the severity of the condition and the type of poultice used.

Removing a poultice should be done gently to avoid any irritation, especially if the skin underneath is tender. Lift the edges of the cloth slowly and wash the area with warm water to remove any residue. It's essential to observe the skin's reaction after removing the poultice and to discontinue use if any adverse effects occur, such as increased redness or irritation.

The cleanup after removing a poultice is straightforward. Any remnants of the poultice can be composted if they're purely organic, while the cloth can be washed and reused. Always store any reusable materials in a clean, dry place to ensure they are ready for next use without any risk of contamination or degradation.

Crafting and applying poultices is a deeply rewarding practice, connecting you to the healing power of nature through direct application of its gifts. As you explore various herbs and their benefits, you'll gain not only relief from specific ailments but also a greater appreciation for the natural remedies available at your fingertips. Whether it's soothing a stubborn rash or easing the pain of a sprain, poultices offer a tangible and potent form of healing that enhances your journey toward natural health.

2.5 Herbal Oils: Preparation for Women's Wellness

In the nurturing world of herbal remedies, infused oils stand out as versatile and potent mediums for harnessing the therapeutic properties of herbs. These oils carry with them the essence of the plants, offering a gentle yet effective way to integrate the healing power of herbs into your daily life. Whether used in massage therapies, skincare formulations, or simply as aromatic compounds, herbal oils blend the ancient tradition of herbal medicine with contemporary needs for health and beauty. Let's explore the enriching process of creating your own herbal oils, tailored to nourish your body and uplift your spirit.

Creating infused herbal oils begins with selecting the right base or carrier oil. Each carrier oil has its own unique properties and benefits, and the choice of oil can signif-icantly influence the therapeutic qualities of your final product. Common carrier oils include olive oil, known for its antioxidant properties and skin-nourishing benefits, making it an excellent choice for general wellness and skin care. Coconut oil, with its rich fatty acid content, offers deep moisturizing benefits and is particularly effective for conditioning hair and skin. For those with a preference for a lighter texture, almond oil is superb, providing a non-greasy feel while still offering substantial moisturizing and softening properties. Jojoba oil is another excellent choice, especially for facial care, as it closely mimics the skin's own sebum (an oily substance that protects your skin from drying out), making it naturally conditioning without clogging pores.

To infuse the oil, begin by gently heating your chosen carrier oil in a double boiler to just below simmering. Then, add dried herbs of your choice - lavender for calming, rosemary for invigorating, or chamomile for soothing. The key is to keep the heat low to preserve the delicate properties of the oil and the herbs. Allow the herbs to steep in the oil for 1-3 hours, depending on how strong you want the infusion. Throughout the process, it's vital to monitor the oil to ensure it does not overheat. Once the infusion process is complete, strain the herbs from the oil using a fine mesh sieve or cheesecloth, squeezing out as much oil as possible. The result is a beautifully infused herbal oil that carries both the scent and the beneficial properties of the herbs.

Herbal oils find their magic in versatility. They can be used as massage oils, offering not only the benefits of the herbs but also the therapeutic touch of massage, which together can enhance circulation and relieve stress. When used in skincare, these oils can be applied directly to the skin or added to homemade lotions or creams to add moisturizing and specific healing properties. For instance, calendula-infused oil can be used on its own or in formulations to help heal dry, irritated skin. For hair care, oils infused with rosemary or nettle can be massaged into the scalp to stimulate hair growth and improve scalp health. Beyond topical applications, these oils can also be used in aromatherapy, with their scents helping to alter mood and support emotional well-being.

Storing your herbal oils properly is crucial to maintain their effectiveness and extend their shelf life. Always store infused oils in airtight containers away from direct sunlight. Dark glass bottles are ideal as they help block light that can degrade the oil. Keep the bottles in a cool, dry place - a cabinet away from heat sources like stoves or heaters is perfect. Properly stored, most herbal oils can last up to one year. If you notice any changes in the smell, color, or texture of the oil, it may be a sign of spoilage, and the oil should be discarded. By taking care with the creation and storage of your herbal oils, you ensure that these natural remedies retain their healing properties and stand ready to support your wellness journey whenever you need them.

2.6 Easy Pills and Capsules for Busy Schedules

In the continuous quest for health optimization, one cannot overlook the practicality and effectiveness of herbal pills and capsules, particularly for those with demanding schedules. Creating your own herbal pills offers a direct, controlled, and convenient way to incorporate the healing benefits of herbs into your daily routine. When you prepare your herbal capsules, you know exactly what's in them and can tailor the combinations to suit your specific health needs without the additives often found in commercial products. This customization not only allows for targeted health solutions but also ensures you are consuming only the highest quality ingredients.

The preparation of herbal pills and capsules begins with assembling a few basic tools and ingredients. You will need high-quality dried herbs, a capsule machine, empty capsules, and possibly a grinder if your herbs are not already finely powdered. The choice of herbs depends on your health goals; for instance, echinacea can be used for boosting the immune system, while valerian root is excellent for promoting sleep and reducing anxiety. It's crucial to source your herbs from reputable suppliers to ensure they are pure, free from contaminants, and sustainably harvested. Once you have your herbs and equipment, you are ready to begin the encapsulation process.

Making herbal pills at home is surprisingly straightforward with the use of a capsule machine, which can typically fill several capsules simultaneously. Start by finely grinding your chosen herbs to a powder - this increases the surface area, making it easier for your body to absorb the beneficial compounds. If you do not have a grinder, a high-powered blender can work in a pinch, though it may not achieve the same fineness. Once your herbs are powdered, follow the instructions specific to your capsule machine: typically, this involves placing the empty capsules into the machine, spreading the herbal powder over them, and then using the machine to close the capsules. This process can be a meditative practice as you focus on the health benefits these capsules will bring to your life.

Dosage and storage are critical aspects of using herbal pills effectively and safely. Determining the correct dosage of herbal capsules can vary based on the herb and your individual health needs. It's wise to start with the lower dosage recommendations and adjust as needed based on your body's response. Consulting with a healthcare provider knowledgeable in herbal medicine can provide guidance tailored to your specific conditions and needs. Once your capsules are prepared, store them in a cool, dry place, ideally in a dark glass bottle to protect them from light, which can degrade the herbs' potency. Properly stored, these capsules can last for several months, ensuring you have a ready supply of your herbal remedies as part of your health regimen.

Incorporating these herbal pills into your daily routine can be seamlessly done. For example, you might take a capsule of milk thistle daily with your breakfast to support liver health or a capsule of ginger before meals to aid digestion. The convenience of herbal capsules allows you to enjoy the benefits of herbs without the preparation time typically involved with teas or tinctures, fitting effortlessly into even the busiest of schedules. This method of using herbal medicine offers you the flexibility and efficiency needed to maintain your health naturally amidst the demands of modern life. By preparing your own herbal pills and capsules, you ensure that you are equipped with natural remedies that are not only tailored to your health needs but also prepared according to the highest standards of purity and potency. As we continue to explore more herbal preparation methods, remember that each technique offers unique benefits and applications, contributing to a holistic approach to wellness that empowers you to take control of your health in a way that fits your lifestyle and preferences.

In wrapping up this chapter on crafting your own herbal remedies, we've journeyed through various methods that harness the intrinsic properties of herbs - from soothing teas and powerful tinctures to protective salves and practical capsules. Each preparation offers unique benefits, whether it's the ritualistic brewing of tea that calms the mind or the convenience of capsules that support health without fuss. The art of creating these remedies opens up a path to greater self-sufficiency and a deeper connection with the healing powers of nature, aligning ancient herbal wisdom with the needs of modern life. As you continue to explore these methods, let each one enrich your understanding and enhance your well-being, paving the way for a healthier, more balanced life. As we move forward, the next chapter will delve into specific herbal remedies tailored to address common health concerns, providing you with practical applications and recipes to integrate into your daily health regimen.

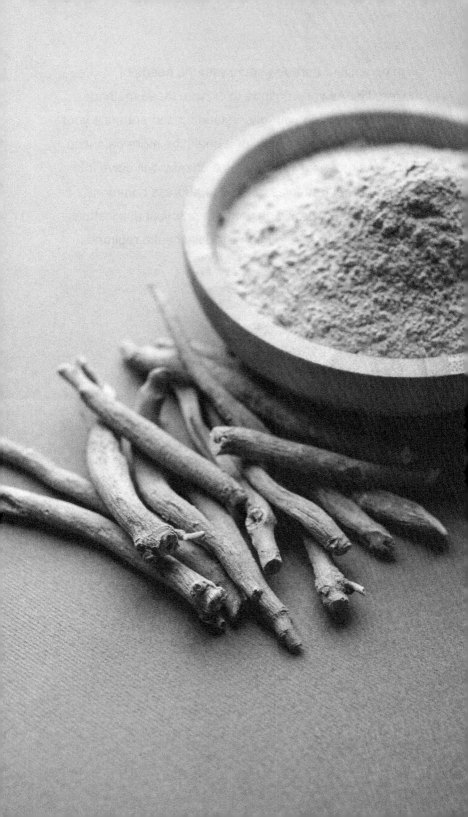

CHAPTER 3
HORMONAL HARMONY

In the delicate dance of daily life, your hormonal health plays a leading role, orchestrating a range of bodily functions from mood regulation to reproductive health. However, when stress and external pressures throw off your hormonal balance, it can feel like your body's own systems are working against you. Fortunately, nature provides a class of herbs known as adaptogens, which act like a skilled conductor, helping to restore harmony and balance to your body's endocrine system. These remarkable herbs support your body's ability to adapt to stress and promote a sense of equilibrium, making them indispensable allies in today's fast-paced world.

3.1 Adaptogens for Stress and Hormonal Balance

Adaptogens are a unique group of herbal ingredients used to improve the health of your adrenal system, the system that manages your body's hormonal response to stress. They help bolster the body's resilience in dealing with both physical and emotional stressors. By supporting adrenal function, adaptogens facilitate balance throughout the endocrine system, enhancing your ability to maintain homeostasis - your body's natural state of balance. The endocrine system is a complex network of glands and organs that uses hormones to control and coordinate your body's metabolism, energy level, reproduction, growth and development, and response to injury, stress, and mood. This ability to stabilize physiological processes and promote homeostasis makes adaptogens a powerful tool in managing stress and optimizing hormonal health. Numbered among the most celebrated adaptogens are ashwagandha, rhodiola, and holy basil, each with unique properties that contribute to their effectiveness in hormonal balance and stress reduction:

- Ashwagandha is renowned for its ability to reduce cortisol levels, the body's stress hormone. It enhances your resilience to stress and helps to stabilize mood swings, making it particularly beneficial for those experiencing stress-related hormonal imbalances.

- Rhodiola not only helps combat fatigue and improve energy levels but also improves cognitive functions that can be impaired by stress. It's particularly effective during stressful times when you need a mental boost.

- Holy basil, also known as tulsi or Queen of Herbs, works by lowering blood cortisol levels and supporting the body's natural detoxification processes. Its calming effect on the nervous system makes it an excellent herb for those who find themselves frequently overwhelmed by the stress of daily life.

Incorporating adaptogens into your daily routine in various forms - teas, tinctures, and capsules - allows you to choose the method that best fits your lifestyle:

- Teas provide a comforting way to ingest adaptogens, ideal for those who enjoy the ritual of drinking tea. A cup of ashwagandha or Holy Basil tea can be a calming addition to your morning or evening routine.

- Tinctures are concentrated herbal extracts that provide a quicker, more potent delivery of adaptogens. They are particularly useful for those needing immediate effects, such as during a stressful day at work.

- Capsules offer a convenient and measured dose of adaptogens, suitable for those with busy lives. They ensure you receive a consistent dose, which can be crucial for long-term hormonal balance.

It's always important to consult with a healthcare provider to determine the appropriate dosage for your specific needs, as adaptogens can vary in potency and effects from person to person.

To illustrate the effectiveness of adaptogens, consider the case of Maria, a 38-year-old mother of two, who struggled with chronic stress and fatigue. Despite her healthy lifestyle, she found herself constantly overwhelmed and irritable, which she attributed to her demanding job and busy family life. After a consultation with a herbalist, Maria began taking a daily regimen of rhodiola rosea in capsule form. Within a few weeks, she noticed a significant improvement in her energy levels and mood. The adaptogen helped modulate her stress response, allowing her to engage with her family more positively and manage her work responsibilities without the usual fatigue and anxiety.

This real-life example underscores the transformative potential of adaptogens in managing stress and restoring hormonal balance. By integrating these natural regulators into your wellness routine, you can reclaim control over your hormonal health, paving the way for a more balanced, vibrant life. As you explore the benefits of ashwagandha and of rhodiola and holy basil, remember that the journey to hormonal harmony is not just about alleviating symptoms but about nurturing a deeper sense of well-being that resonates through every aspect of your life.

3.2 Managing PMS Naturally with Herbs

Navigating the monthly ebb and flow of premenstrual symptoms (PMS) can often feel like an unwelcome rollercoaster ride for many women. From bloating and mood swings to debilitating cramps, PMS can significantly impact your quality of life. However, nature offers a treasure trove of herbal allies that can help manage these symptoms more gently and effectively. Herbs such as chaste tree berry (Vitex) and dong quai have been revered for centuries in traditional medicine for their ability to bring balance and relief during the menstrual cycle.

Chaste tree berry, particularly, is lauded for its effectiveness in normalizing hormone-induced imbalances. It works primarily on the pituitary gland, which controls the release of luteinizing hormone (LH), a chemical in your body that triggers important processes in your reproductive system. By promoting the production of LH, Vitex indirectly enhances progesterone production, which is often low during PMS. This adjustment can alleviate symptoms like breast tenderness and mood fluctuations. Dong quai, often referred to as 'female ginseng,' complements this by promoting blood flow to the pelvis, which helps soothe cramps and other menstrual irregularities.

For those who experience bloating, a common yet uncomfortable PMS symptom, dandelion tea can be a simple, natural diuretic that helps the body eliminate excess fluid. To prepare, steep one teaspoon of dried dandelion root in boiling water for 10 minutes. This tea not only alleviates water retention but also provides potassium, which can be lost when taking synthetic diuretics. For mood swings and irritability, consider a calming cup of lemon balm tea, which acts as a mild sedative and helps to improve mood and reduce anxiety.

Creating tinctures from these herbs can also offer concentrated relief. A simple tincture might combine chaste tree berry and dong quai to balance hormones and support overall reproductive health. To make this, macerate the dried herbs in a jar with a high-proof alcohol like vodka, ensuring the herbs are completely submerged. Seal the jar and store it in a cool, dark place, shaking daily for four to six weeks before straining. This tincture can be taken in small doses, typically 1-2 ml, in the morning to help stabilize hormonal levels throughout the day.

Integrating these herbal remedies into your daily life doesn't have to be a daunting task. It begins with a mindful approach to your body's rhythms and signals, allowing you to anticipate and mitigate symptoms before they become disruptive. Start by tracking your menstrual cycle and noting when you typically experience PMS symptoms. This awareness can help you determine the best times to begin incorporating herbal remedies, ideally a week or two before symptoms usually start. Adding these herbs to your daily regimen can be as simple as replacing your morning coffee with a cup of dandelion or lemon balm tea. For those on the go, capsules containing Vitex or dong quai offer a convenient way to ensure consistent dosage without having to prepare teas or tinctures daily. Incorporating these into your morning routine after breakfast can help promote optimal absorption and effectiveness.

Moreover, consider the holistic benefits of combining these herbs with dietary adjustments. Increasing intake of calcium and magnesium-rich foods, such as leafy greens and nuts, can enhance the effectiveness of herbal treatments by supporting muscle relaxation and nervous system function. Similarly, reducing intake of salt and caffeine can help minimize bloating and irritability, common culprits during PMS.

Embracing a holistic approach to managing PMS involves more than just treating symptoms as they arise; it encompasses a lifestyle that supports hormonal health continuously. Regular exercise, for example, can significantly alleviate PMS symptoms by improving circulation and releasing endorphins, which naturally boost mood and pain tolerance. Yoga and gentle aerobic exercises like walking or cycling can be particularly beneficial.

In addition to physical activity, stress management plays a crucial role in holistic PMS care. Techniques such as meditation, deep breathing exercises, or journaling can help manage stress levels, thereby reducing the severity of PMS symptoms. Integrating these practices during your premenstrual phase can make a noticeable difference in how you experience and manage PMS.

Ultimately, the confluence of herbal remedies, proper nutrition, regular exercise, and effective stress management creates a comprehensive strategy that not only addresses the symptoms of PMS but also enhances your overall health and well-being. This proactive and inclusive approach ensures that you are equipped to manage PMS naturally and effectively, minimizing its impact on your life and allowing you to embrace each phase of your cycle with grace and vitality.

3.3 Herbs for Fertility and Reproductive Health

In the beautiful quest to nurture life, understanding and optimizing your reproductive health can play a pivotal role. Nature offers a plethora of herbs known for their remarkable ability to enhance fertility and support overall reproductive wellness. Among these, red clover and nettle leaf stand out for their profound efficacy. Red clover is rich in isoflavones, a type of phytoestrogen (plant estrogen) that can play a crucial role in improving hormonal balance and promoting uterine health, which are vital for conception. Nettle leaf, on the other hand, is laden with iron and vital minerals, supporting not only the health of the uterus but also preparing the body for the increased demand for nutrients during pregnancy. For those in the pre-conception phase, focusing on creating an optimal internal environment is essential. Herbs can be instrumental in this process, particularly through their ability to detoxify and prepare the body for pregnancy. Milk thistle, with its potent silymarin compound (antioxidant with anti-inflammatory properties), supports liver health, crucial for balancing hormones and clearing toxins from the body. Dandelion root complements this by promoting healthy kidney function and aiding in the elimination of waste and excess hormones. These herbs work synergistically, not just detoxifying the body but also nourishing it, creating a fertile ground for new life.

The nutritional aspect of herbs should not be overlooked in the context of fertility and reproductive health. Herbs like raspberry leaf are highly esteemed not only for their pleasant flavor but also for their high vitamin and mineral content, which are crucial during the pre-conception and pregnancy periods. Raspberry leaf is particularly revered for its high levels of magnesium, potassium, iron, and b-vitamins, which are vital for both mother and baby. It is often recommended as a uterine tonic because of its ability to strengthen the muscles of the pelvic region, potentially making for an easier and healthier pregnancy and delivery.

Incorporating these fertility-enhancing herbs into your daily regimen can be both delightful and beneficial. For instance, starting your day with a tea blend of red clover and nettle can invigorate and prepare your body with essential nutrients. Alternatively, a capsule form of milk thistle or dandelion root can be a practical way to ensure consistent daily intake, crucial for their cumulative benefits. Furthermore, creating a ritual around taking these herbs - perhaps a quiet moment in the morning with a cup of raspberry leaf tea - can not only be nourishing but also provide a moment of reflection and connection with your body's natural rhythms.

Moreover, integrating these practices with a balanced diet rich in whole foods, regular exercise, and stress-reducing techniques like yoga or meditation can amplify the effects of the herbs, creating a holistic approach to fertility. Remember, the path to enhancing fertility is as much about nurturing the body and mind as it is about the specific treatments or herbs you choose to use. Each step taken is a step towards creating a welcoming, healthy environment for new life, and the journey itself can be as nurturing as the goal.

3.4 Menopause: Herbal Allies for Transition

Menopause marks a significant phase in a woman's life, characterized by the end of menstrual cycles and a series of physiological changes that can affect physical, emotional, and mental well-being. Common symptoms such as hot flashes, night sweats, mood swings, and sleep disturbances can be challenging. However, the gentle power of herbal remedies offers considerable relief and support during this transition. Understanding which herbs effectively alleviate specific menopausal symptoms can empower you to manage this natural life stage with more ease and comfort.

Hot flashes and night sweats are perhaps the most commonly mentioned symptoms of menopause, often making day-to-day life uncomfortable. Fortunately, herbs like black cohosh and sage have been shown to provide significant relief. Black cohosh in particular, has been extensively studied for its effectiveness in reducing the frequency and intensity of hot flashes. It functions by acting as a phytoestrogen; plant-based compounds that mimic the effects of estrogen in the body, helping to balance hormone levels gently. This action can alleviate not only hot flashes but also other symptoms associated with hormonal fluctuations during menopause. To integrate black cohosh into your regimen, consider starting with a standardized extract, which can provide consistent dosing. It's typically available in tincture or capsule form, making it easy to incorporate into your daily routine.

Sage, another invaluable herb during menopause, offers relief from night sweats and can reduce overall body perspiration. Its natural astringent properties help calm excessive sweating, a common annoyance during menopause that can disrupt sleep and daily activities. Sage tea is a simple and effective way to harness these benefits. Steeping fresh or dried sage leaves in boiling water for about 5 to 10 minutes not only yields a potent medicinal drink but also provides a moment of tranquility during your day. Drinking a cup of sage tea in the evening can help reduce night sweats and promote a more restful sleep.

Emotional fluctuations, including mood swings and irritability, are also common as the body adjusts to changing hormone levels during menopause. St. John's Wort and lemon balm are excellent for stabilizing mood and enhancing emotional well-being. St. John's Wort is particularly known for its antidepressant properties and can be very effective in lifting mood and alleviating depression often associated with menopause. However, it's important to consult with a healthcare provider before starting St. John's Wort, as it can interact with several medications. Lemon balm, on the other hand, acts as a mild sedative and can help calm nerves and ease anxiety. It is delightful when consumed as a tea and can be paired with other herbs like lavender to enhance its relaxing effects.

Creating a personalized menopause herbal regimen involves understanding not only which herbs are beneficial but also how best to use them to suit your unique needs. Start by identifying the symptoms that are most disruptive to your life and then select herbs known to alleviate those specific issues. For instance, if sleep disturbances and night sweats are your primary concerns, you might focus on integrating sage and black cohosh into your evening routine. On the other hand, if mood swings and anxiety are more pressing, incorporating St. John's Wort and lemon balm throughout your day could be beneficial.

When designing your regimen, consider the form in which you take these herbs. Teas and tinctures are wonderful for their ease of use and the ability to combine multiple herbs for a synergistic effect. Capsules may be better suited for those who prefer convenience and precise dosing. It is also wise to think about how these herbs fit into your daily schedule. For example, a calming herbal tea might be perfect for your bedtime routine, while a capsule could be more convenient during a busy workday.

Lastly, remember that lifestyle factors play a crucial role in managing menopause symptoms effectively. Regular exercise, a balanced diet rich in phytoestrogens (plant nutrients found in several different types of food such as soy products, grains, beans, and some fruits and vegetables), calcium and good hydration are all crucial. Coupling these practices with your herbal regimen not only helps alleviate menopausal symptoms but also supports overall health and wellness during this transformative phase. As you adjust and refine your approach based on your body's responses, you will find a rhythm and routine that not only eases the symptoms of menopause but also enhances your quality of life during these years. It is important to note that while some herbal treatments for menopause are compatible with HRT, if you are having treatment for or have previously been treated for estrogen-based cancers, herbal supplements should only be adopted under the supervision of a healthcare provider.

Some of the most common herbal supplements can interfere with anti-hormonal agents used for breast cancer. If you are taking tamoxifen or have had estrogen-based cancer in the past, you should avoid red clover, St. John's Wort, black cohosh and licorice, as they may affect your hormone levels and the efficacy of your treatment. As with any serious medical condition, please consult a healthcare provider before adding any herbal remedies to your regimen.

3.5 Thyroid Health: Herbal Remedies and Support

The thyroid gland, a small butterfly-shaped organ located in the front of your neck, plays a crucial role in regulating numerous metabolic processes throughout the body. It produces hormones, primarily thyroxine (T4) and triiodothyronine (T3), which influence metabolism, body temperature, growth and development. Disruptions in thyroid function can lead to significant health issues, with common conditions being hypothyroidism, where the gland underproduces thyroid hormones, and hyper-thyroidism, an overproduction of these hormones. Symptoms of hypothyroidism include fatigue, weight gain, and sensitivity to cold, whereas hyperthyroidism may cause weight loss, high levels of anxiety, tremors, and heat intolerance. Managing thyroid health is thus essential for maintaining overall well-being and metabolic balance.

Among the herbal remedies beneficial for thyroid health, bladderwrack and ashwagandha stand out due to their adaptogenic and nutrient-rich profiles. Bladderwrack, a type of seaweed, is a natural source of iodine, a critical nutrient for thyroid function. Iodine plays a pivotal role in the synthesis of thyroid hormones, and its deficiency can lead to hypo-thyroidism. Incorporating bladderwrack into your diet can help ensure adequate iodine levels, thereby supporting normal thyroid function. Clinical studies have shown that the intake of bladderwrack has been associated with the normalization of thyroid-stimulating hormone (TSH) levels, especially in individuals with mild iodine deficiency. However, it is crucial to use this herb under supervision, as excessive iodine can also disrupt thyroid function.

Ashwagandha, another powerful herb, supports the thyroid gland by modulating the release of stress hormones, which can adversely affect thyroid health. It helps to enhance the conversion of T4 to the more active T3, thus improving symptoms of hypothyroidism. A 2017 study published in the "Journal of Alternative and Complementary Medicine" found that ashwagandha improved serum thyroid hormone levels, suggesting its benefits for people with thyroid dysfunction. Integrating ashwagandha into your wellness routine, either in capsule form or as a tea, can aid your body's ability to maintain hormonal balance and resilience against stress.

Maintaining thyroid health extends beyond herbal supplements; it encompasses a holistic approach involving diet and lifestyle adjustments. A thyroid-supportive diet includes foods rich in selenium, zinc and antioxidants, which are vital for thyroid hormone production and protection of the thyroid gland from oxidative stress. Foods such as Brazil nuts, shellfish, and eggs are excellent sources of selenium, while zinc can be found in high concentrations in pumpkin seeds and lentils. Antioxidant-rich fruits and vegetables, like berries and spinach, should also be staples in your diet to help reduce oxidative stress, which is often elevated in thyroid disorders. Stress management is another critical component.

Chronic stress can lead to an imbalance in adrenal hormones like cortisol, which can interfere with thyroid hormone production and utilization. Incorporating regular stress-reducing practices such as yoga, meditation, or deep-breathing exercises can significantly improve your body's ability to regulate hormones effectively. In addition, ensuring adequate sleep is vital, as sleep deprivation can exacerbate hormonal imbalances, including those involving the thyroid.

While herbal remedies can significantly support thyroid health, it is very important to monitor their effects through regular blood tests that assess hormone levels and thyroid function. This monitoring allows you to adjust dosages or change your approach based on concrete physiological feedback. For instance, if you are taking bladderwrack for its iodine content, keeping track of your thyroid hormone levels can help prevent the potential for iodine-induced hyper-thyroidism. Similarly, regular check-ins with a healthcare provider can ensure that any herbal supplementation aligns with other treatments and overall health needs.

It is also important to be aware of how your body feels and to notice any changes in symptoms. For example, if you observe a reduction in fatigue or a stabilization of weight while using ashwagandha, these could be tangible indicators of its positive impact. Conversely, any new or worsening symptoms should prompt a re-evaluation of your current herbal regimen and possibly a consultation with your healthcare provider. This proactive approach not only maximizes the benefits of herbal remedies but also ensures your thyroid health is managed safely and effectively, supporting your overall well-being in a balanced and informed manner.

3.6 Boosting Libido: Herbs for Sexual Health

In exploring herbal medicine, one cannot overlook the role of natural aphrodisiacs in enhancing sexual health and vitality. Herbs such as maca, tribulus, and shatavari not only support sexual function but also enrich your overall quality of life by boosting libido and enhancing energy levels. Maca, a root native to the Andes, is known for its remarkable effect on energy, stamina, and sexual function in both men and women. It works by balancing hormone levels and can particularly invigorate those who feel drained or stressed. Tribulus, often used in traditional practices across different cultures, has been shown to support libido and sexual function, particularly in men, by increasing the levels of certain hormones that are linked to sexual desire. Shatavari, celebrated in Ayurvedic medicine (Ayurveda "knowledge of life" is an alternative medicine system with historical roots in the Indian sub-continent - heavily practiced in India and Nepal) as a potent tonic for women, nourishes the female reproduc-tive system and helps to balance hormones, which can enhance sexual desire and overall vitality.

The importance of a holistic approach to sexual health cannot be overstated. This approach encompasses not only the physical aspects of sexual function but also the emotional and psychological components that contribute to a fulfilling sex life. Stress, anxiety, and emotional dis-connect can significantly dampen sexual desire and satis-faction. By integrating herbs that support both emotional well-being and physical health, you can create a more balanced foundation for your sexual health. For example, incorporating ashwagandha alongside sexual health-specific herbs can help manage stress and anxiety, thereby enhancing your overall readiness and response to sexual activity. This holistic method ensures that you are not just treating symptoms but nurturing a more vibrant, energetic, and balanced self.

Creating an enchanting atmosphere with herbal recipes can also play a significant role in enhancing romance and intimacy. Consider the simple yet profound act of sharing a cup of herbal tea made from damiana, a herb known for its aphrodisiac properties, which can set a tone of warmth and connection. Alternatively, a massage oil infused with sensual herbs like ylang-ylang and rose can heighten the tactile experience, deepening intimacy and affection. Preparing a blend is straightforward: mix a few drops of these essential oils with a carrier oil such as sweet almond or jojoba oil, and use it to lovingly massage your partner, fostering not only physical closeness but also emotional presence.

While exploring herbal remedies to boost libido and enhance sexual health, it is crucial to prioritize safety, consent, and open communication. Every individual's body reacts differently to herbs, and what works for one person may not work for another or might even cause adverse reactions. Therefore, starting with small doses and observing how your body responds is key to safely integrating new herbs into your regimen. Furthermore, discussions about sexual health and preferences with your partner are essential. This open dialogue ensures that both parties feel comfortable and consensual in their exploration of herbal aphrodisiacs and other methods to enhance intimacy. Remember, the cornerstone of a fulfilling sexual relationship is mutual respect and clear communication, ensuring that all interactions are consensual and joyously agreed upon.

This exploration of herbs for boosting libido and enhancing sexual health invites you to consider not only the physical benefits of such natural remedies but also the deeper, relational aspects they can nurture. By integrating these herbs into your life, you invite a holistic enhancement of your health, where sexual well-being is interlinked with emotional and physical vitality, each element supporting and enhancing the other. As you continue to explore the potential of herbal remedies to enrich your life, let the principles of safety, consent, and open communication guide your journey, ensuring that your exploration enhances both your own well-being and the health of your relationships.

Moving forward, the subsequent chapter will delve into the realm of herbal remedies for mental and emotional well-being, exploring how natural treatments can support cognitive function, alleviate stress, and elevate mood, continuing our exploration of how herbal medicine can enhance every facet of your health and life. This natural progression from physical and sexual health to mental and emotional care highlights the interconnectedness of our bodily systems and the holistic nature of herbal medicine.

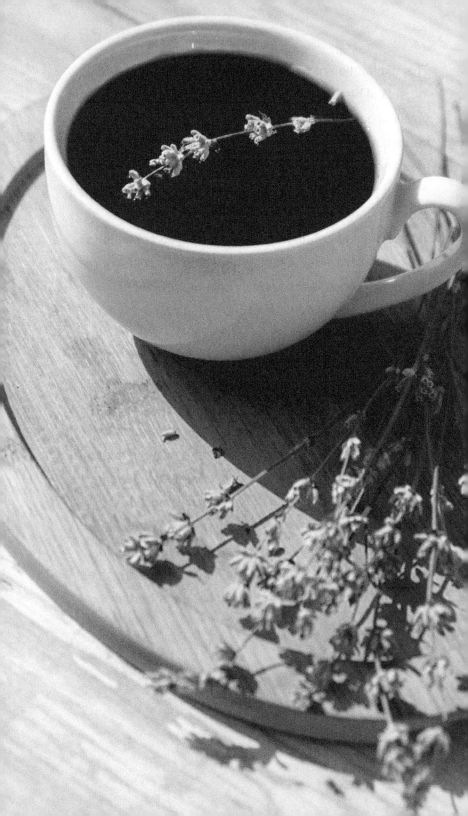

CHAPTER 4
MENTAL AND EMOTIONAL WELLBEING

Navigating the complexities of modern life often leaves little room for personal reflection and mental rest, making it all too easy for stress and anxiety to take hold. Understanding how to soothe your mind and to fortify your emotional resilience is not just beneficial; it's a necessity for maintaining your overall health and happiness. This chapter focuses on natural ways to cultivate mental peace and emotional stability using herbal remedies, integrating these ancient practices into your contemporary life ensures a balanced approach to mental wellness.

4.1 Calming the Mind: Herbs for Anxiety and Stress

In times of stress and uncertainty, turning to nature's pharmacy can be remarkably soothing. Herbs such as lavender, chamomile, and passionflower have been used for centuries to help calm the mind and ease the spirit. Lavender, with its sweet, floral aroma, is widely acclaimed for its ability to reduce anxiety and induce relaxation. Its compounds interact with GABA, helping to quieten the nervous system and lower stress responses. Gamma-aminobutyric acid (GABA) is a neurotransmitter, or chemical messenger in the brain. Potential benefits of GABA include lowering blood pressure, reducing muscle spasms and managing mood. Chamomile, often consumed as a gentle, soothing tea, contains apigenin, an antioxidant that binds to certain receptors in the brain that may promote sleepiness and reduce insomnia, which is often a byproduct of anxiety. Passionflower, another powerful herb, boosts the brain's levels of gamma-aminobutyric acid, which lowers brain activity and can help you feel more relaxed.

Creating a calming tea or tincture can be a comforting ritual, bringing a sense of peace to your day. A simple tea recipe might include a blend of chamomile and lavender, combined in equal parts. Steep one teaspoon of this blend in hot water for about ten minutes to unleash its full calming potential. For those who might benefit from something stronger, a tincture combining passionflower and valerian root offers a potent remedy. Mix one part passionflower to one part valerian root in a jar, cover with vodka, and let sit for four weeks, shaking daily. This tincture can be taken in small doses, especially during periods of heightened stress, to effectively soothe the mind and reduce anxiety.

To deepen your relaxation and enhance the effects of herbal remedies, consider pairing them with practices like yoga and meditation. For instance, sipping a cup of chamomile tea before a meditation session can prepare your mind for deep relaxation. Alternatively, diffusing lavender oil during a yoga practice can enhance the calming atmosphere, making it easier to release tension and stress. These combinations allow for a holistic approach to stress management, addressing both the physical and psychological aspects of anxiety.

While herbal remedies provide significant relief from mild to moderate anxiety, they are part of a broader spectrum of treatment options. It's crucial to recognize their limits. Severe cases of anxiety often require professional intervention and possibly medical treatment. Herbs can support these treatments but should not replace them. If you find that your anxiety is not improving or is getting worse, it's important to reach out to a mental health professional. They can offer guidance tailored to your specific needs, which may include integrating herbal remedies alongside other therapeutic options.

To deepen your understanding of what triggers your stress and how you respond, consider keeping a reflective journal. Regularly jot down what situations trigger your anxiety and how you feel physically and emotionally. This practice can not only provide insights into patterns and triggers but also help you track the effectiveness of the herbal remedies and relaxation techniques you are using. Over time, this journal can become a valuable tool in managing your stress and enhancing your emotional well-being.

4.2 Herbal Sleep Tonics for Insomnia

In addressing the silent epidemic of insomnia that many face, the natural world offers solace not just through silence but through sleep-promoting herbs like valerian root and hops. Valerian root, revered for its sedative qualities, can significantly shorten the time it takes for you to fall asleep and enhance the quality of sleep you enjoy. Its active compounds interact with GABA receptors in the brain, a mechanism similar to that of synthetic sedatives, without the unwanted side effects. Hops, commonly known for its role in brewing beer, contains naturally occurring compounds that also promote sleep and work well in conjunction with valerian. Together, they form a powerful duo that can help ease the body into a restful night without the grogginess often associated with chemical sleep aids.

Establishing a bedtime ritual is another transformative strategy that can enhance your sleep quality. This ritual can include the brewing and consumption of a sleep-promoting herbal tea. Imagine ending your day with a warm cup of tea made from a blend of hops and valerian root, perhaps with a hint of lavender or chamomile to enhance the flavor and soothing effects.

The process of preparing the tea itself can be a calming prelude to sleep, signaling to your body that it's time to wind down. Additionally, consider incorporating aroma-therapy into your bedtime routine. Essential oils such as lavender or bergamot can be used in a diffuser; their soothing scents fill your bedroom, creating a tranquil environment conducive to sleep.

When using sedative herbs like valerian root and hops, it's important to understand and practice safe usage. These herbs are generally safe for most people when used in moderation. However, reliance on any sleep aid, natural or not, should be carefully managed. It's advisable to use these herbs as part of a broader strategy to manage insomnia rather than as a sole solution. This approach ensures that you aren't developing a dependency but rather using the herbs to support other healthy sleep practices. If you find yourself needing to use these herbs regularly, it might be a signal to evaluate other underlying causes of your sleep disturbances, possibly with the help of a healthcare professional.

Incorporating good sleep hygiene practices alongside herbal remedies can dramatically improve their effectiveness. This includes maintaining a regular sleep schedule, ensuring your bedroom is conducive to sleep (think cool, dark, and quiet), and limiting exposure to screens and bright lights in the hour leading up to bedtime. Perhaps you could read a book or engage in light stretching or meditation instead of screen time right before bed. By creating an environment and routine that signals to your body that it's time to sleep, you enhance the natural effects of the herbal tonics, making it easier to drift off and stay asleep through the night. As you integrate these practices and remedies into your life, remember that the goal is to support and enhance your body's natural sleep processes. The combination of herbal remedies with thoughtful sleep hygiene practices offers a holistic approach to conquering insomnia, helping you to wake refreshed and ready to meet the challenges of your day. This integrated approach not only improves your nights but enriches your overall well-being, proving that a good night's sleep is a cornerstone of health.

4.3 Uplifting Herbs for Depression and Mood Swings

In the pursuit of emotional stability and mental health, it's vital to recognize the role of nature in shaping our mood and well-being. Certain herbs have been identified not just for their physical health benefits but for their profound impact on mental health, particularly in alleviating symptoms of depression and stabilizing mood swings. St. John's Wort, rhodiola, and saffron are among those that have been researched and celebrated for their mood-enhancing properties. These herbs offer a beacon of hope for many who prefer natural treatment methods, providing a complementary approach to traditional therapies.

St. John's Wort, for instance, has a rich history of use in herbal medicine for treating depression. It contains active compounds such as hypericin and hyperforin, which are thought to have neurotransmitter-modulating effects. Its mechanism, similar to many antidepressants, includes the inhibition of the reuptake of certain neurotransmitters such as serotonin and dopamine, thus increasing their availability in the brain. This action can significantly elevate mood and alleviate depressive symptoms. Multiple clinical studies validate the efficacy of St. John's Wort in treating mild to moderate depression. A meta-analysis of studies published in the "Cochrane Systematic Review" found it to be more effective than a placebo and as effective as standard anti-depressant medications for mild to moderate depression, yet with fewer side effects.

Rhodiola is another robust herb known for its adaptogenic properties, helping the body resist various stressors. It works by enhancing the sensitivity of neurons to the presence of dopamine and serotonin, two neurotransmitters involved in the regulation of mood, focus, and overall emotional well-being. This makes rhodiola particularly effective not only in alleviating depressive symptoms but also in boosting cognitive functions and combating fatigue, which are often associated with depression.

Clinical trials, including a study published in the "Nordic Journal of Psychiatry," showed that patients with mild-to-moderate depression who took rhodiola experienced significant improvements in various symptoms, including insomnia, emotional stability, and somatization, without serious side effects. Somatization is the expression of psychological or emotional factors as physical (somatic) symptoms. For example, stress can cause some people to develop headaches, chest pain, back pain, nausea or fatigue.

Saffron, often dubbed the "sunshine spice," not only adds vibrant color and flavor to dishes but is also a powerful mood enhancer. Its antidepressant properties may be attributed to safranal and crocin, compounds that are believed to modulate neurotransmitters in a similar way to certain antidepressants. Research, including randomized controlled trials, suggests that saffron can improve symptoms of depression at doses of about 30 mg per day. A review published in the "Journal of Integrative Medicine" highlighted several studies where saffron not only improved mood but was also found to be as effective as some conventional medications used for treating mild to moderate depression.

Integrating these herbs into a comprehensive approach to mental health involves more than just consuming them; it requires a holistic strategy that includes dietary adjustments, physical activity, and possibly other therapeutic interventions. For those seeking to incorporate these herbs into their daily routine, it is recommended to start with teas or supplements, following dosage guidelines provided by trustworthy sources or healthcare providers. St. John's Wort, for example, can be taken as a daily supplement, with studies suggesting doses ranging from 300 to 600 mg to be effective. However, due to its interaction with various medications including birth control pills and certain antidepressants, it's crucial to consult with a healthcare provider before starting any regimen involving St. John's Wort. Rhodiola can be consumed in capsule or tea form, ideally in the morning to utilize its energizing effects throughout the day. Saffron can be easily incorporated into meals or taken as a supplement.

It's equally important to recognize when professional help is needed. While these herbs can provide significant relief, they are not a substitute for professional medical treatment in cases of severe depression. Consulting with a healthcare provider can help determine the best treatment plan, which might include a combination of herbal remedies, conventional medications and other therapies. This integrative approach not only ensures safety but also maximizes the potential for successful management of symptoms, supporting your journey toward better mental health and emotional balance.

4.4 Focus and Clarity: Herbs for Cognitive Support

In the pursuit of mental clarity and enhanced cognitive function, the natural world offers some remarkable allies. Ginkgo biloba, gotu kola, and rosemary are not just plants; they are gateways to improved focus, memory retention, and overall brain health. Each of these herbs carries unique properties that make them potent cognitive enhancers, suitable for inclusion in your daily regimen to support brain health and mental performance.

Ginkgo biloba has long been revered for its ability to improve blood circulation, which is crucial for optimal brain function. By increasing blood flow to the brain, ginkgo biloba helps enhance the oxygen and nutrient supply needed for cognitive processes, thereby improving concentration and memory. Its rich content of flavonoids and terpenoids, known for their strong antioxidant effects, also helps protect the brain from neuronal damage and diseases. Gotu kola, known as the "herb of longevity," supports cognitive function differently. It is believed to enhance the body's ability to produce collagen, which fortifies the veins and capillaries that supply blood to the brain. This not only improves the brain's oxygen supply but also helps in detoxifying the body, which can improve mental clarity and longevity. Rosemary, with its delightful aroma, contains carnosic acid, an antioxidant that fights off free radical damage in the brain. The inhalation of rosemary essential oil has been shown to increase the concentration of neurotransmitters that boost mood and mental clarity. It must be noted though, that because rosemary can increase blood pressure, consumption isn't suitable for those with hypertension, ulcers, Crohn's disease or ulcerative colitis. High doses should also be avoided in pregnancy.

The concept of herbal nootropics takes these natural cognitive enhancers to the next level. Nootropics, substances that can improve cognitive function, particularly executive functions, memory, creativity, or motivation, in healthy individuals, are not new. However, the use of herbs as nootropics offers a holistic approach to cognitive enhancement that aligns with the body's natural processes. For instance, combining ginkgo biloba and gotu kola can provide a synergistic effect, enhancing not only memory and focus but also increasing resilience to mental stress and anxiety. This combination helps maintain cognitive functions in high-pressure situations, providing a natural boost to perform tasks that require mental endurance and sharpness.

Integrating these cognitive-supporting herbs into your daily routine can be both enjoyable and effective. Start your day with a morning tea infused with rosemary and gotu kola to kickstart your brain functions. Alternatively, consider a mid-morning tincture of ginkgo biloba, which can be taken with water or a drink of your choice. This not only ensures that you receive their benefits throughout the day but also helps in establishing a consistent routine that supports cognitive health. For those who might forget to take their herbs in the morning rush, setting reminders or preparing your doses in advance can be a useful strategy to ensure you do not miss out on these cognitive benefits.

However, it's crucial to balance herbal cognitive enhancement with adequate rest and mental exercises. Just as the body needs physical activity to stay fit, the brain requires challenges to maintain its cognitive faculties. Simple activities like solving puzzles, learning a new skill, or engaging inregular intellectual discussions can stimulate brain function and enhance the efficacy of herbal nootropics. Equally, ensuring sufficient sleep each night allows the brain to consolidate memory and repair neuronal damage, which is essential for maintaining the cognitive benefits gained from herbal nootropics. In this way, a balanced approach not only enhances immediate cognitive functions but also contributes to long-term brain health and mental acuity.

As you explore these herbal solutions for enhancing cognitive function, consider the seamless integration of these herbs into your lifestyle as an investment in your mental acuity and overall well-being. Whether through teas, tinctures, or essential oils, these herbs offer a natural, effective way to boost cognitive function and support a vibrant, healthy mind.

4.5 Aromatherapy for Emotional Balance

Aromatherapy, the therapeutic use of essential oils extracted from plants, offers a profound way to enhance emotional and psychological well-being. Oils such as lavender, bergamot, and ylang-ylang are particularly effective in influencing mood and emotions, each bringing its own unique essence and benefits to the spectrum of emotional health. Lavender, renowned for its soothing qualities, is a go-to for reducing stress and promoting a sense of calm. Its sweet, floral scent is believed to activate the brain's limbic system, which is involved in emotion regulation, thus helping to soothe anxiety and foster relaxation. Bergamot, with its bright, citrus aroma, can help alleviate stress and improve mood. It's often used in treatments for depression as it can stimulate the production of dopamine and serotonin, leading to feelings of freshness and joy. Ylang-ylang, known for its rich, floral fragrance, is used to elevate mood and alleviate stress, tension, and irritability. Its ability to enhance emotional equilibrium makes it invaluable in aromatherapy blends aimed at emotional balance.

Exploring the different methods of using these essential

oils can significantly enhance their effectiveness. One of the most popular methods is through the use of diffusers, which disperse the essential oil molecules into the air, allowing for easy inhalation and continuous benefits. Diffusing lavender in your living space in the evenings can help unwind your mind after a busy day, promoting relaxation before bedtime. For those facing a challenging day ahead, diffusing bergamot in the morning can invigorate the senses and boost mood. Alternatively, topical application of these oils, when diluted with a carrier oil like almond or coconut, can be just as effective. Massaging a few drops of ylang-ylang mixed with a carrier oil onto your wrists or the back of your neck can provide direct, soothing effects and help stabilize mood swings throughout the day.

Creating personalized blends of these oils allows for targeted approaches to managing emotional health. Start by identifying what emotional state you wish to support or transform. For instance, if you're seeking to reduce stress and promote relaxation, you might create a blend combining lavender for its calming properties, bergamot for its mood-lifting effects, and ylang-ylang for its ability to ease mind chatter. Begin with equal parts of each, adjusting based on which scent you prefer and how your body responds. It's essential to mix these oils in a small glass bottle, adding a carrier oil if you plan to use them topically. Experimenting with the ratios and combination can be a delightful process, leading you to a formula that resonates perfectly with your emotional and aromatic preferences.

However, while the benefits of aromatherapy are vast, it is crucial to approach its practice with an awareness of safety and sensitivity. Essential oils are highly concentrated and can be potent, necessitating careful handling. Always perform a patch test on a small area of skin before using an oil topically to ensure there is no adverse reaction. If diffusing oils, make sure the room is well-ventilated, particularly if asthma or other respiratory issues are a concern. Be mindful of the potency of the oils; a few drops are often sufficient, especially when starting. Overuse can lead to sensitivity or even an adverse reaction. Consulting reputable sources or professionals on proper dilutions and applications can safeguard against potential risks, ensuring that your aromatherapy experience enhances your well-being without unintended consequences.

Navigating the aromatic world of essential oils offers a pathway to greater emotional health that is as enriching as it is fragrant. Whether diffused, applied topically, or blended to perfection, these oils carry the essence of nature's therapeutic powers, ready to soothe, uplift, and balance your emotional landscape. As you integrate these natural essences into your daily routine, their subtle yet profound effects can help steer your emotional well-being towards a more balanced and joyful state, enhancing your quality of life in the most natural way.

4.6 Creating a Calming Herbal Bath Experience

Imagine stepping into a warm, fragrant bath, where the stresses of the day begin to melt away as the soothing properties of natural herbs envelop you. Creating this serene experience is not just an indulgence; it's a potent therapeutic practice that can significantly enhance your mental and physical well-being. The tradition of herbal baths, known for their profound ability to calm the mind and soothe the body, integrates the therapeutic virtues of water with the healing presence of herbs and essential oils.

Selecting the right herbs and essential oils is crucial for crafting a bath that not only relaxes but also rejuvenates. Epsom salts, known for their high magnesium content, serve as an excellent base for any herbal bath, aiding in muscle relaxation and stress reduction. To this, adding herbs like eucalyptus, known for its refreshing and decon-gesting properties, can transform your bath into a revital-izing retreat, especially beneficial if you're feeling under the weather. For a more soothing herbal bath, consider rose petals and chamomile. Rose petals, rich in antioxi-dants and aromatically luxurious, offer skin-soothing prop-erties and emotional uplift. Chamomile, on the other hand, is celebrated for its calming effects on the skin and the nervous system, making it perfect for an evening soak.

Crafting an effective herbal bath blend involves more than just tossing herbs into hot water. A thoughtful combination can enhance the therapeutic benefits and create a more enjoyable experience. For a stress-relieving bath, a blend of lavender, chamomile, and a few drops of frankincense oil can be ideal. Lavender promotes relaxation, chamomile soothes, and frankincense adds a grounding, comforting note that deepens the calming effects. To prepare, fill a small cloth bag with equal parts of dried lavender and chamomile flowers, add a few drops of frankincense essential oil, and tie it securely. Hang this sachet under the faucet as you run your bath, allowing the hot water to cascade through the herbs, releasing their essences.

The ritual of bathing itself holds therapeutic potential that goes beyond cleanliness. Submerging in warm water can help lower cortisol levels, easing the symptoms of stress and anxiety. The warmth increases blood flow and relaxes muscles, while the herbs contribute their healing properties through your skin and inhalation. To elevate this experience into a holistic self-care ritual, consider the ambiance of your bathing environment. Soft lighting, perhaps from candles, can add a gentle glow that enhances relaxation. A soft, instrumental playlist can also complement the serene atmosphere, helping you to disconnect from the outside world and engage more deeply with the sensations of the bath.

Enhancing your bath with additional elements like music, candles, and a cup of herbal tea can transform it into a truly multisensory experience. For instance, playing a selection of soft, ambient tunes can help soothe your mind, while candles provide a soft, flickering light that encourages relaxation.

Sipping on a warm cup of herbal tea made from pepper-mint or lemon balm can amplify the internal benefits of your herbal bath, aiding in digestion and further promoting relaxation from within. This combination of external and internal herbal therapy not only maximizes the relaxation potential but also turns your bath into a comprehensive healing session, addressing both mind and body.

As you integrate these practices and elements into your bathing ritual, you create not just a method for cleansing but a transformative routine that nurtures both your physical and emotional well-being. This ritualistic approach to bathing serves as a gentle reminder of the importance of taking time for yourself, encouraging a deeper connection to your senses and inner peace. Whether it's by soothing sore muscles, offering a moment of tranquility, or providing a sensory escape from stress, a well-crafted herbal bath can be a foundational practice in your self-care regimen, fostering resilience and also serenity in your everyday life.

As we conclude this exploration into the soothing world of herbal baths, remember that the art of bathing is as much about nurturing the spirit as it is about cleansing the body. Each element, from the herbs you select to the environment you create, contributes to a holistic experience that can restore balance and renew vitality. This practice, steeped in both tradition and personal care, not only enriches your life but also deepens your connection to the natural world. With each bath, you're invited to steep in the restorative powers of herbs, emerging refreshed and realigned.

Looking ahead, the next chapter will delve into the world of digestive health, exploring how herbs can play a pivotal role in enhancing digestive function and overall gut health. Just as herbal baths cleanse and comfort the external body and soothe the mind, herbal remedies for digestion help purify and optimize your internal processes, ensuring that your journey toward holistic health is as comprehensive as it is natural.

UNLOCK THE POWER OF GENEROSITY

MAKE A DIFFERENCE WITH YOUR REVIEW

"The best things in life come from helping others, even if we don't see the results." - Unknown

Isn't it amazing how doing something nice for someone else can make you feel great? That's because people who help others tend to be happier. So, let's try something together. Do you remember what it was like when you first started learning about herbal remedies? Maybe you were a bit confused and looking for some guidance. That's how others feel right now, and you can help them!

I wrote HERBAL REMEDIES FOR BUSY WOMEN because I want everyone to know how rewarding and easy it can be to use herbs to improve health. But I need your help to reach as many people as possible. Most people choose a book based on its cover and what others say about it. That's why I'm asking if you could leave a review. It won't cost you anything and takes less than a minute, but your words could change someone's life.

Your review could help more women feel empowered to take charge of their health naturally, more families learn to use herbal remedies at home and more people feel confident in choosing healthier options. Spread the joy and benefits of natural remedies to others.

Here's how you can leave your review (it's super easy!):

Scan the QR code below to go directly to the review page:

Think of it this way: if you help someone today by sharing your thoughts on this book, you're part of a wonderful chain of kindness.

If you feel good about helping, then you're definitely my kind of person! Welcome to our community of caring, health-conscious individuals. I can't wait to share more about the power of herbs in the chapters to come.

Thank you from the bottom of my heart for your kindness and generosity and for joining me on this journey.

Your biggest fan, *Luna*

PS - Remember, when you offer something valuable, like a helpful review, you become valuable to others. If you think this book can help another busy woman like you, why not share it with her too?

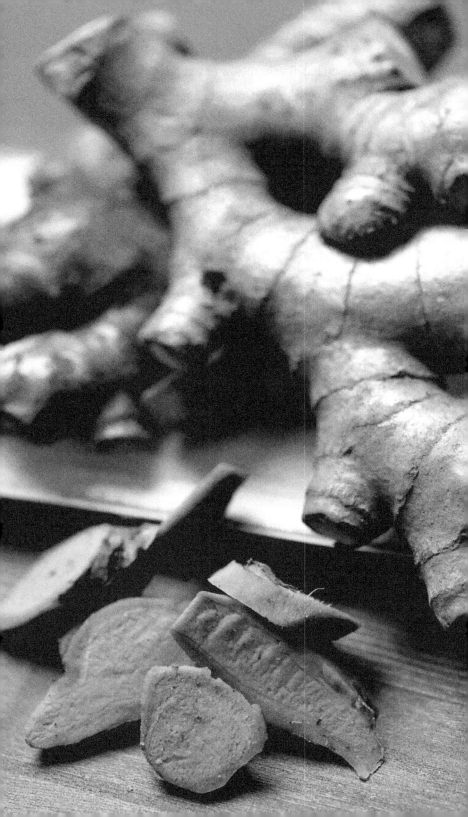

CHAPTER 5
DIGESTIVE HEALTH

N avigating the complexities of digestive health can
often seem as intricate and personal as the foods we
choose to eat. Just as a well-balanced meal can invigorate and sustain us, understanding how to nurture our
digestive system with herbal remedies promises not only
comfort but also a deeper harmony within our bodies.
In this chapter, we explore gentle, effective herbs that
soothe and support digestion, helping to transform this
everyday process into a cornerstone of holistic health.

5.1 Gentle Herbs for Digestive Upset

Digestive discomfort is a common ailment that can disrupt
one's day and can often be a sign that our bodies are out
of sync with what we consume or how we live.
Fortunately, nature offers a palette of gentle herbs such
as peppermint, ginger, and fennel, each renowned for
their soothing properties that can help calm an upset
stomach and enhance digestive harmony. Peppermint,
with its natural antispasmodic properties, is excellent
for relieving symptoms like gas and bloating. It works by

relaxing the smooth muscles of the digestive tract, easing the discomfort that often accompanies indigestion. Ginger, a revered spice across various cultures, is celebrated not only for its robust flavor but also for its ability to stimulate saliva, bile, and gastric juice production, which aids in the digestion of food. Its warming effect is particularly beneficial in alleviating nausea and vomiting. Fennel, with its distinctive licorice-like flavor, contains compounds that can help reduce inflammation and relax the muscles in the gastrointestinal tract, making it a valuable ally against bloating and cramps.

Herbal teas not only warm and comfort the soul but also serve as potent remedies for digestive issues. Crafting a tea blend using the herbs mentioned can be both therapeutic and enjoyable. For instance, a simple digestive tea can be made by steeping 1 teaspoon of dried peppermint leaves, ½ teaspoon of grated fresh ginger, and ½ teaspoon of fennel seeds in boiling water for 10 minutes. This blend not only soothes the stomach but also stimulates digestion, making it a perfect after-meal beverage. For those experiencing nausea, a ginger tea made by simmering fresh ginger slices in water for about 15 minutes can be particularly effective. Adding a touch of honey not only enhances the flavor but also offers additional soothing benefits.

Integrating these digestive herbs into daily meals not only

enhances the flavors of the dishes but also fortifies digestive health proactively. Ginger, for instance, can be grated
into stir-fries or boiled into soups, lending its piquant
flavor and digestive benefits. Fennel seeds can be toast-
ed and sprinkled over salads or incorporated into breads
and pastries, offering a crunchy, healthful boost.
Peppermint leaves make a refreshing addition to iced
teas or can be chopped and added to desserts for a cool,
soothing finish. Regularly including these herbs in your
meals can help maintain digestive efficiency and prevent
discomfort before it starts.

While herbal remedies offer significant benefits, it's crucial
to recognize when digestive symptoms may require
professional evaluation. Persistent symptoms such as
severe abdominal pain, significant and unintentional
weight loss, recurrent nausea or vomiting, or changes in
bowel habits could signal underlying health issues that
necessitate medical intervention. Understanding these
signs and responding promptly by consulting healthcare
professionals ensures that greater complications can be
avoided, and appropriate treatments can be administered.
This proactive approach, coupled with the supportive
nature of herbal remedies, provides a comprehensive
strategy for maintaining optimal digestive health.

To further enhance your understanding and management
of digestive health, consider maintaining a reflective

journal focused on your digestive well-being. Regularly record what you eat, any symptoms of discomfort, and how you feel both physically and emotionally after meals. Over time, this journal can help you identify patterns or specific foods that may be contributing to digestive issues, allowing you to make informed adjustments to your diet or lifestyle. Additionally, note any improvements observed from incorporating herbal remedies into your routine. This practice not only fosters a deeper connection with your body's digestive processes but also empowers you to take proactive steps towards lasting digestive health and overall well-being.

5.2 Detoxifying Herbs for Liver Health

The liver, your body's primary detoxification organ, plays a pivotal role not only in filtering toxins but also in metabolizing nutrients, balancing hormones, and supporting overall vitality. This remarkable organ is constantly at work, managing everything from cholesterol levels to blood sugar. To support its myriad functions, certain herbs stand out for their liver-cleansing properties, acting as natural allies in maintaining liver health and enhancing detoxification processes. Milk thistle, dandelion, and turmeric are among those celebrated for their effective support of liver function, each bringing unique benefits to this essential organ.

Milk Thistle, scientifically known as Silybum marianum, contains silymarin, a group of compounds touted for their antioxidant and anti-inflammatory properties. Silymarin not only protects liver cells from damage by acting as an anti-oxidant but also promotes liver regeneration. It has been widely studied for its efficacy in treating liver diseases such as hepatitis and cirrhosis, as well as for protecting the liver from potential toxins, including those found in alcohol and certain medications. Dandelion, often perceived merely as a persistent weed, has roots and leaves that are potent detoxifiers. Dandelion promotes liver detoxification by supporting bile production and flow, essential for breaking down fats and helping to purge waste products from the body. Moreover, its diuretic properties assist in eliminating toxins by increasing urine production, thereby reducing the strain on the liver.

Turmeric, a vibrant spice known for its deep golden color, offers significant benefits for liver health through curcumin, its active ingredient. Curcumin is celebrated for its potent anti-inflammatory and antioxidant effects. It helps in reducing liver inflammation and protecting against liver injury by minimizing the effects of harmful toxins. This is particularly beneficial in preventing the build-up of fats within the liver, a condition known as fatty liver disease, which can lead to more severe liver issues if left unchecked.

To harness the benefits of these herbs, creating a liver detox blend can be both a therapeutic and proactive approach to liver health. To prepare a simple yet effective herbal detox tea, combine one part milk thistle seeds, one part dandelion root, and half part turmeric root. Gently crush the milk thistle seeds to release their active compounds. Simmer all ingredients in water for about 15 minutes to extract their beneficial properties. Straining this mixture will yield a potent tea that can be consumed twice daily to aid liver detoxification. For those who prefer a more convenient option, capsules containing standardized extracts of these herbs can also be effective, ensuring you receive their benefits in a controlled, measurable way.

Incorporating these detoxifying herbs into your lifestyle involves more than just consuming them; it also means fostering habits that support your liver's health. Diet plays a crucial role in this. Foods rich in antioxidants, such as leafy green vegetables, berries, nuts, and seeds, can enhance the liver's ability to detoxify the body effectively. Reducing the intake of processed foods, sugars, and unhealthy fats is equally important, as these can strain the liver and impede its functioning. Regular physical activity and maintaining a healthy weight also contribute significantly to liver health, helping to prevent conditions like fatty liver disease, which can impair the liver's ability to function optimally.

Mindful consumption of alcohol and medications, and avoiding exposure to environmental toxins wherever possible, are crucial steps in protecting your liver. Remember, the liver's capacity to detoxify is not limitless. By supporting it with the right herbs and lifestyle choices, you are not only enhancing its functionality but also reinforcing your overall health and well-being. Engaging in regular check-ups can also help monitor liver health, especially if you have a history of liver disease or are exposed to factors that may compromise liver function. This proactive approach ensures that your liver continues to perform its essential tasks, supporting your health seamlessly as you navigate the complexities of life.

5.3 Herbal Teas for Bloating and Gas Relief

Addressing the discomforts of bloating and gas often requires a gentle, yet effective approach, and the world of herbal remedies offers a treasure trove of natural solutions that can alleviate these common digestive issues. Chamomile and caraway stand out among these solutions, not only for their efficacy but also for their availability and ease of use. Chamomile, widely appreciated for its calming effects on the mind, also works wonders on the digestive system. Its anti-spasmodic properties help relax the muscles of the digestive tract, which can relieve the discomfort of gas and bloating. Caraway seeds, on the other hand, are known for their carminative properties, which promote the expulsion of gas and prevent the formation of new gas, thereby easing bloating and creating a soothing effect on the stomach.

Creating a blend of these herbs in a tea can be particularly beneficial. When blending herbs for tea to alleviate bloating and gas, it's important to consider both the medicinal properties of the herbs and the balance of flavors. To create a soothing, effective tea, you might start with a base of chamomile, known for its gentle, apple-like flavor, and add caraway seeds for their slightly spicy, earthy notes. This combination not only enhances the tea's ability to relieve digestive discomfort but also creates a pleasantly aromatic and flavorful beverage. To prepare the tea, add one teaspoon of dried chamomile flowers and a half teaspoon of crushed caraway seeds to a cup of boiling water. Let it steep for 10 minutes before straining. This allows for optimal extraction of both the soothing compounds and the flavors.

Timing and dosage are crucial for maximizing the benefits of this herbal tea. For best results, it's advisable to drink the tea after meals, especially if you've consumed foods that you know tend to cause bloating and gas. This timing helps the body manage the digestive processes more efficiently, using the natural properties of the herbs to prevent discomfort before it starts. As for dosage, while these herbs are generally safe for regular use, it's recommended to start with one cup of tea after meals and observe how your body responds. You can adjust the strength of the tea or the frequency of consumption based on your specific needs and the results you experience.

Incorporating dietary changes can also significantly enhance the effectiveness of these herbal teas. A diet high in fiber can sometimes contribute to increased gas production, so balancing fiber intake with other nutrients and observing how your body responds can be beneficial. Additionally, reducing the intake of artificial sweeteners, carbonated drinks, and high-fat foods, which can exacerbate bloating and gas, might also help. Instead, focus on including probiotic-rich foods like yogurt, kefir, and fermented vegetables, which support digestive health and can improve the overall effectiveness of the herbal remedies you are using. By combining these dietary adjustments with the consumption of chamomile and caraway tea, you create a comprehensive approach to managing bloating and gas, enhancing your digestive health with every meal. This holistic approach, blending the benefits of herbal teas with thoughtful dietary practices, not only addresses the symptoms of bloating and gas but also contributes to a more robust digestive health strategy. As you continue to explore and integrate these practices into your daily routine, you may find a significant improvement in how you feel after eating, turning mealtime back into a source of nourishment and pleasure rather than discomfort.

5.4 Maintaining a Healthy Gut Flora with Herbs

Understanding the significance of gut health is central to appreciating why nurturing our intestinal flora is so pivotal to overall wellness. Prebiotics, a type of dietary fiber, play a crucial role in this process. They act as food for probiotics, the beneficial bacteria residing in our gut, helping these microbes thrive and flourish. Among the natural sources of prebiotics, herbs like chicory and dandelion root stand out for their high inulin content, a potent pre-biotic fiber. Inulin not digested or absorbed in the stomach but stays in the bowel and helps certain beneficial bacteria to grow. It is a starchy substance found in a wide variety of fruits, vegetables, and herbs, including wheat, onions, bananas, leeks, artichokes, and asparagus. Chicory, with its rich history as a coffee substitute, is more than just a beverage alternative; it is a powerful gut health enhancer. The inulin in chicory promotes the growth of beneficial gut bacteria, which in turn can improve digestion, enhance the absorption of minerals, and boost the immune system. Similarly, dandelion root, often utilized for its detoxifying properties, contains inulin which not only supports the liver but also fosters a healthy gut environment. These roots can be incorporated into your diet in various forms such as teas, powders, or even as a cooked vegetable, offering a versatile and effective way to enhance your gut flora.

Fermentation is a transformative process, not only for foods and beverages but also for maximizing the health benefits of herbs. Fermented herbal drinks, enriched with probiotics, can effectively enhance gut health by introducing beneficial bacteria that aid in digestion and improve nutrient absorption. Preparing these beverages can be an enjoyable and rewarding practice. For instance, creating a fermented dandelion and burdock drink involves simple ingredients and steps that can be easily followed at home. Start by brewing a strong herbal tea using dandelion and burdock roots, known for their cleansing properties and beneficial effects on the liver and gut. Once the tea is ready, add a natural sweetener like honey, which acts as a fuel for the fermentation process. Introduce a starter culture such as a water kefir or a probiotic capsule to begin the fermentation and allow the mixture to ferment in a glass jar for a few days. The result is a probiotic-rich herbal drink that supports digestive health and enhances your gut flora.

The health of our gut is inextricably linked to numerous aspects of our overall health, including our immune system, mental health, and chronic disease risk. A balanced gut microbiota is essential not only for optimal digestion but also for the synthesis of necessary vitamins and the regulation of the immune system. When our gut flora is balanced, we are better protected against pathogens, more capable of absorbing nutrients from our food, and less likely to suffer from autoimmune diseases and chronic inflammations. Moreover, recent studies have illuminated the connection between gut health and mental health, suggesting that a healthy gut might contribute to a more stable mood and lower anxiety levels. This connection, often referred to as the gut-brain axis, highlights the profound impact that our gut health can have on our mental and emotional well-being, underscoring the importance of maintaining a healthy gut through diet, lifestyle, and the judicious use of beneficial herbs. Incorporating gut-supportive herbs into your daily diet can be both simple and effective. For instance, adding freshly grated ginger to your meals can aid digestion and help reduce inflammation, thanks to its powerful compounds like gingerol. Turmeric, another potent herb, can be incorporated into your diet by adding it to smoothies, curries, or teas. Its active compound, curcumin, is not only anti-inflammatory but also enhances bile production, which is crucial for the digestion and absorption of fats. For those looking to increase their intake of prebiotic-rich herbs, adding raw or lightly cooked chicory and dandelion greens to salads or soups can be an excellent way to boost your inulin intake, fostering a healthy gut environment. To ensure these practices become a consistent part of your lifestyle, consider setting aside a little time each week to prepare and store these herbs in ways that make them easily accessible and simple to incorporate into your daily meals. This ongoing commitment to nurturing your gut health will support your overall wellness, keeping your digestive system - and indeed, your entire body - in optimal condition.

5.5 Fighting Inflammation with Turmeric and Ginger

In the realm of natural health, turmeric and ginger stand out not only for their distinct flavors but also for their powerful anti-inflammatory properties, making them indispensable in the management of digestive health and beyond. Turmeric, a vibrant yellow spice, is lauded for its compound curcumin, which has been extensively studied for its profound anti-inflammatory effects. Curcumin helps modulate the body's inflammatory processes through its ability to inhibit key enzymes and cytokines (signaling proteins that help control inflammation in your body) that contribute to inflammation. This action is particularly beneficial in the digestive tract, where chronic inflammation can lead to conditions such as inflammatory bowel disease (IBD) and irritable bowel syndrome (IBS). Ginger, with its sharp, invigorating flavor, contains gingerols, shogaols, and paradols, compounds known for their anti-inflammatory and antioxidant properties. These compounds work synergistically to soothe inflamed tissues within the digestive system, helping to reduce bloating, cramps, and other discomforts often associated with digestive disturbances.

The therapeutic use of turmeric and ginger extends to their ability to enhance the integrity of the stomach lining and to promote the healing of gastric and peptic ulcers. By reducing inflammation, these spices help to protect the stomach cells against the corrosive effects of gastric acids. This protective action not only helps to alleviate current digestive discomfort but also aids in preventing future digestive issues. Moreover, the antioxidant properties of both turmeric and ginger play a crucial role in neutralizing free radicals within the gastro-intestinal tract, which can contribute to inflammation and cell damage. This aspect is especially important considering the potential link between chronic inflammation and various gastrointestinal cancers. By incorporating these spices into your diet, you not only enjoy their flavor but also leverage their protective qualities against digestive inflammation and related health issues. Integrating turmeric and ginger into your daily meals can be a delightful and healthful practice. One simple way to incorporate these spices is through a daily anti-inflammatory tea. To prepare this, slice a small piece of fresh ginger and add it to a pot with a teaspoon of turmeric powder and a cup of water. Let it simmer for about 10 minutes, allowing the flavors and properties to infuse the water. Strain the mixture into a cup and add a teaspoon of honey and a squeeze of lemon juice for flavor. This tea can be a comforting, warming beverage that soothes the digestive system and combats inflammation.

For a more substantive incorporation, consider a turmeric-ginger stir-fry. Begin by heating a tablespoon of coconut oil in a pan, adding a teaspoon each of freshly grated ginger and turmeric as the oil warms. Add your choice of vegetables, such as bell peppers, broccoli, and carrots, and stir-fry until they are just tender. The spices will coat the vegetables, infusing them with flavor and anti-inflammatory properties. Serve this stir-fry over a bed of brown rice or quinoa for a nourishing meal that supports digestive health and overall well-being. Another creative way to enjoy these spices is through a turmeric-ginger marinade, ideal for chicken, fish, or tofu. Combine a tablespoon each of turmeric and ginger powder with garlic, a bit of olive oil, lemon juice, and salt to taste. Coat your protein choice in the marinade and let it sit for at least an hour before cooking. This not only flavors the food but also imparts the anti-inflammatory benefits of the spices, making your meal both delicious and therapeutic. The efficacy of turmeric and ginger in combating inflammation is supported by numerous scientific studies, underscoring their role in holistic health practices. Research published in the Journal of Medicinal Food highlights how curcumin, the active compound in turmeric, significantly lowers levels of inflammatory markers in the blood. These findings are corroborated by clinical trials that demonstrate curcumin's ability to improve symptoms of inflammatory conditions like rheumatoid arthritis and inflammatory bowel disease, showcasing its broad-spectrum anti-inflammatory properties.

Similarly, studies on ginger have identified its potential to reduce inflammation at a cellular level. Research in the Journal of Pain reports that daily ginger consumption results in moderate-to-large reductions in muscle pain following exercise-induced muscle injury. This effect is attributed to ginger's ability to inhibit the production of pro-inflammatory cytokines; proteins that tell immune cells where to go and what to do to keep your immune system functioning correctly and chemokines, which direct immune cells toward places in your body where they can fight infection. These proteins provide a natural and effective way to manage inflammation and associated pain.

To maximize the anti-inflammatory effects of turmeric and ginger, it is beneficial to adopt complementary lifestyle practices that support overall inflammatory health. Main-taining a diet rich in other anti-inflammatory foods such as omega-3 fatty acids, found in fish like salmon and in flaxseeds, can enhance the effects of turmeric and ginger. Additionally, incorporating regular physical activity into your routine can help to further reduce inflammation throughout the body. Activities such as yoga and swimming not only promote physical fitness but also reduce stress, which can be a significant contributor to systemic inflammation.

Ensuring adequate sleep and hydration are also crucial for managing inflammation. Sleep allows the body to repair and regenerate, helping to reduce inflammation, while staying hydrated helps to flush toxins from the body, further reducing inflammatory responses. By integrating these practices with the regular consumption of turmeric and ginger, you can create a comprehensive anti-inflammatory regimen that supports your digestive health and enhances your overall quality of life.

5.6 Herbal Remedies for Food Sensitivities

Food sensitivities can often be elusive and manifest through various digestive discomforts such as bloating, gas, diarrhea, and even fatigue or headaches. Unlike food allergies, which trigger the immune system and can cause severe reactions, food sensitivities involve a more gradual reaction and can be harder to pinpoint. The first step in addressing these sensitivities is to identify the specific foods that cause discomfort. This often involves keeping a detailed food diary where you document everything you eat and note any symptoms that follow. Over time, patterns can emerge that suggest which foods might be troubling your digestive system. For a more structured approach, you might consider an elimination diet, which involves removing common irritants like dairy, gluten, soy, and added sugars from your diet for a period, then gradually reintroducing them one at a time to observe reactions.

To soothe the digestive tract irritated by food sensitivities, herbs such as slippery elm and marshmallow root are invaluable. Slippery elm contains mucilage, a substance that becomes a slick gel when mixed with water. This gel coats and soothes the mouth, throat, stomach, and intestines,making it an excellent remedy for irritation in the gastro-intestinal tract.

Similarly, marshmallow root also contains high levels of mucilage and offers soothing properties that can relieve irritation and inflammation in the digestive system. Both herbs can be taken as a tea or in capsule form. To prepare a soothing tea, simply steep one teaspoon of the powdered herb (slippery elm or marshmallow root) in boiling water for a few minutes and drink it two to three times a day, especially before meals.

Managing food sensitivities effectively extends beyond identifying triggers and soothing symptoms; it involves a comprehensive dietary management strategy. An elimination diet is often helpful in this regard, as it involves removing suspected foods from your diet and then methodically reintroducing them to see how your body reacts. It's crucial during this process to maintain a balanced diet to ensure you still receive necessary nutrients. This might involve working with a nutritionist to find suitable alternatives to excluded foods. Moreover, during the reintroduction phase, integrating digestive aids such as herbal teas made from ginger or peppermint can help manage minor reactions and support digestion. Building digestive resilience is about strengthening the entire digestive system so it can handle occasional irritations without significant discomfort. This involves regular intake of digestive-supportive herbs and adopting practices that generally support digestive health. For instance, daily consumption of herbal teas that promote digestion and soothe the digestive tract can be a foundational practice. Practices such as eating smaller, more frequent meals, ensuring adequate hydration, and engaging in regular physical activity can significantly enhance your digestive system's resilience. Over time, these practices can help reduce the frequency and intensity of reactions to food sensitivities, leading to improved digestive health and overall well-being. In summary, managing food sensitivities involves a multi-faceted approach that includes identifying potential triggers, using herbal remedies to soothe the digestive system, and adopting a comprehensive dietary management strategy. Through careful observation and intentional dietary choices, supplemented by beneficial herbal remedies like slippery elm and marshmallow root, you can alleviate the discomfort associated with food sensitivities and enhance your digestive health.

As we close this chapter on digestive health, we reflect on the intricate dance of diet, herbs, and practices that support a robust digestive system - a cornerstone of overall health. Each step taken to identify irritants, soothe the system, and strengthen resilience contributes to a more vibrant, energetic life, free from the discomforts of digestive upset. Looking ahead, the next chapter will explore the rejuvenating world of natural skincare, where herbs play a pivotal role in enhancing beauty naturally and sustainably. This transition from internal to external care underscores the holistic approach of herbal remedies, enhancing not just our health but also our natural beauty.

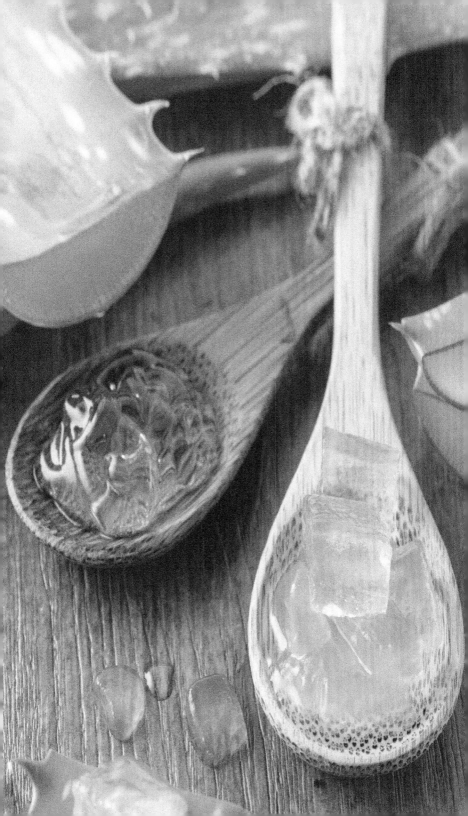

CHAPTER 6
SKIN AND HAIR CARE

S tepping into the realm of skin care, quite often, the simplest secrets to radiance are nestled in nature's lap. This chapter is dedicated to transforming your skin care routine into a nurturing ritual that not only enhances your skin's natural glow but also connects you to the earthy roots of herbal wisdom. Here, the spotlight shines on herbs like aloe vera, chamomile, and turmeric, each celebrated not just for their beauty but for their profound ability to rejuvenate and heal the skin. Through understanding these herbs and integrating them into your daily practices, you embark on a path that not only beautifies but also fortifies your skin against the daily stresses it encounters. Remember, always test a small patch of skin first when applying any mixture to check for allergic reaction.

6.1 Herbs for Glowing Skin: Masks and Scrubs

Aloe vera, chamomile, and turmeric are more than just ingredients; they are staples in the lexicon of natural skin care, each bringing a unique set of benefits. Aloe vera, a gel-filled plant, is renowned for its soothing, moisturizing, and healing properties. It helps in treating sunburn, reducing skin inflammation, and providing a hydrating treat to the skin without leaving a greasy feel. Chamomile, with its anti-inflammatory and antioxidant qualities, is a boon for those with sensitive skin. It calms skin irritations and can lighten your complexion naturally. Turmeric, rich in curcumin, a compound with powerful anti-inflammatory and antioxidant properties, brightens the skin, improves the skin's complexion and rejuvenates dull skin by stimulating new cell growth.

Creating your own herbal face masks allows you to harness the direct benefits of these herbs tailored to your skin type. For a soothing and hydrating mask, blend fresh aloe vera gel with a spoonful of honey. This mask can be applied twice a week for deep hydration. For those with sensitive skin, a chamomile mask can be made by infusing chamomile tea in warm water, mixing it with oatmeal to form a paste. This mixture soothes and reduces redness and is ideal for weekly use. For a brightening effect, mix turmeric powder with yogurt and a few drops of lemon juice to create a mask that reduces pigmentation and evens out skin tone. Apply this mask once a week to witness a gradual illumination of your natural complexion.

Exfoliation is key to removing dead skin cells and rejuvenating the skin's surface. However, it's essential to use gentle scrubs that do not damage the skin. A mix of ground oatmeal, finely ground almonds, and turmeric can serve as an excellent exfoliating scrub that is gentle yet effective. The oatmeal soothes the skin, almonds provide the gentle abrasive texture that sweeps away dead skin cells, and turmeric adds its anti-inflammatory and brightening effects. Use this scrub once a week by gently massaging it in circular motions on your face and neck, followed by rinsing with warm water. Integrating these herbal treatments into your regular skin care routine enhances their effectiveness and benefits.

Consistency is key - using these herbal masks and scrubs as part of your weekly skin care regimen can lead to noticeable improvements over time. For instance, designate one day a week as your "spa day" at home, where you can apply a face mask in the evening, perhaps as you unwind after a bath. Incorporate the exfoliating scrub into your routine every other week, followed by the application of a hydrating aloe vera gel. This not only ensures that you are regularly taking care of your skin but also turns skin care into a therapeutic activity, giving you a chance to relax and pamper yourself, reconnecting with nature's rhythm and your own.

To help you visualize and plan your herbal skin care routine, consider creating a simple chart that schedules when and how to use each herb-based product throughout the week. This could include columns for each day of the week and rows for different types of treatments - masks, scrubs, and moisturizers. Fill in the chart with your chosen treatments, such as "Tuesday: chamomile mask," "Friday: turmeric and oatmeal scrub," and "Daily: aloe vera moisturizer." This visual planning tool can help you maintain consistency and ensure that your skin receives the full spectrum of benefits from these wonderful herbal remedies.

6.2 Natural Solutions for Acne and Eczema

When addressing chronic skin conditions like acne and eczema, turning to nature's bounty offers not just relief but also a gentle, sustainable approach. In particular, witch hazel and tea tree oil are noteworthy for their significant anti-inflammatory and antibacterial properties, making them ideal candidates for your natural skin care arsenal. Witch hazel, derived from the bark and leaves of the Hamamelis virginiana plant, has been used for centuries in traditional medicine due to its potent astringent qualities. It works by tightening skin tissue, easing inflammation, and soothing irritations, making it particularly effective for acne-prone skin. Tea tree oil, extracted from the leaves of the Melaleuca alternifolia tree, native to Australia, contains terpinen-4-ol, a compound with strong antibacterial and antifungal properties. This makes it exceptionally effective in treating acne, as it can penetrate the skin, disinfect pores, and dry out whiteheads, black-heads, and pimples.

Creating topical treatments using these herbs can significantly enhance their effectiveness. For acne, a simple yet powerful topical application can be made by diluting tea tree oil with a carrier oil such as jojoba or sweet almond oil; this mixture can then be applied directly to the affected areas using a clean cotton swab. This method helps in targeting the lesions directly and can prevent the spread of acne-causing bacteria. For eczema, a soothing lotion can be created using witch hazel as the base. Mix this with aloe vera gel and a few drops of lavender essential oil for its calming and anti-inflammatory effects. Applied gently to eczema-affected areas, this blend can help reduce redness, calm itching, and promote healing.

Beyond topical applications, internal support through herbal detoxification plays a crucial role in managing skin conditions like acne and eczema, which are often exacerbated by toxins and impurities within the body. Herbs such as burdock root and milk thistle are renowned for their detoxifying properties. Burdock root helps to purify the bloodstream and improve circulation, thus helping to eliminate toxins from the body. It contains powerful antioxidants, such as quercetin and luteolin, which can also help reduce inflammation and bacterial growth on the skin. Milk thistle supports liver function, a crucial organ for detoxification. It helps to cleanse the body of accumulated pollutants and hormones that can contribute to skin flare-ups. Integrating these herbs into your diet can be as simple as taking them in capsule form or brewing a tea from dried burdock root, which can be enjoyed daily to maintain skin health from the inside out. Preventative measures and maintenance are key in managing skin health and preventing future outbreaks. For individuals prone to acne and eczema, maintaining a regular cleaning routine with gentle, non-irritating products is essential. Avoid harsh facial scrubs or towels that can damage or irritate the skin. Instead, opt for soft washcloths and pat the skin dry gently. Moisturizing is also crucial, even for acne-prone skin; choose non-comedogenic moisturizers that do not clog pores. Regularly changing pillowcases and towels and avoiding touching the face with unwashed hands can also significantly reduce the risk of flare-ups. In your diet, focus on anti-inflammatory foods rich in omega-3 fatty acids, antioxidants, and vitamins, which can support skin health. Foods to avoid include dairy and high glycemic index foods that can trigger or worsen acne and eczema.

Incorporating these practices into your daily life not only addresses the symptoms of these skin conditions but also enhances your overall skin health, leading to a clearer, more radiant complexion. By understanding and utilizing the natural properties of witch hazel and tea tree oil, and supporting your body's internal environment through herbal detoxification, you create a comprehensive approach to skin care that not only treats but also helps to prevent the recurrence of skin issues. This holistic approach ensures that you are not only treating the symptoms but also addressing the root causes of skin conditions, promoting lasting health and vitality of your skin.

6.3 Herbs for Healthy Hair Growth and Strength

When considering the health of your hair, it's essential to look beyond external treatments and focus on the nourishment that fuels its growth from within. Herbs like horsetail and nettle emerge as frontrunners in this category, brimming with vital nutrients that fortify hair from the root to the tip. Horsetail, one of the oldest plants on Earth, is rich in silica, a mineral known for its ability to strengthen hair strands and improve their texture. It also enhances blood circulation to the scalp, which ensures that your hair follicles are nourished with the essential minerals and vitamins they need to produce healthy hair. Nettle, on the other hand, is laden with iron and vitamins A and C, which are crucial for maintaining the health of the scalp and hair follicles. These nutrients not only curb hair loss but also stimulate hair growth by revitalizing the scalp and ensuring the optimal function of the hair growth cycle.

Incorporating these herbs into your hair care routine can be done through dietary supplements or topical applications. For example, creating a hair rinse that includes horsetail and nettle can be particularly effective. You can brew a strong tea with these herbs by steeping them in boiling water for about 20 minutes. Once cooled, this concoction can be used as a final rinse after your regular shampooing routine. This method allows the silica from horsetail and the rich nutrients from nettle to penetrate the scalp and strengthen the hair follicles directly, promoting healthier and more robust hair growth.

Exploring the realm of herbal hair rinses and oils opens up a pathway to naturally lustrous and strong hair. These preparations not only enhance the natural beauty of your hair but also imbue it with the strength and vitality it needs to withstand daily stresses. A rinse made from rosemary and lavender, for instance, can significantly improve hair thickness and growth. Rosemary acts to enhance circulation to the scalp, which increases blood flow and promotes faster hair growth. Lavender, known for its soothing properties, helps in reducing scalp inflammation and dandruff, creating a healthier environment for hair growth.

To create this rinse, you can simmer rosemary and lavender in water for about 15 minutes, strain the mixture, and let it cool. After shampooing, pour this herbal infusion through your hair as a final rinse, gently massaging it into the scalp to stimulate blood flow. For a more potent effect, combining these herbs in an oil infusion can provide deeper nourishment. Warm a carrier oil like coconut or jojoba oil and add dried rosemary and lavender. Let the mixture sit in a warm place for about a week, shaking it daily. This oil can be applied to the scalp and hair a few hours before washing or used as a leave-in treatment for dry ends, offering a sustained release of nutrients.

A healthy scalp is the bedrock of healthy hair growth. Conditions like seborrheic dermatitis, psoriasis, and fungal infections can impede hair growth by affecting the health of the scalp. Herbs such as tea tree and thyme offer powerful antifungal and antibacterial properties that help in treating these scalp conditions. Tea tree oil, for instance, can be diluted with a carrier oil and massaged into the scalp to alleviate symptoms of dandruff and scalp psoriasis. Thyme, with its strong antiseptic properties, can be used in a similar fashion or added to shampoos and conditioners to maintain scalp health.

Creating a scalp treatment with these herbs involves mixing several drops of tea tree and thyme oil with a soothing carrier oil like almond or olive oil. Apply this mixture to the scalp, gently massaging in circular motions to enhance absorption and blood flow. Let it sit for at least an hour or overnight before washing out. Regular use of this treatment can significantly reduce scalp issues, thereby creating a healthier base for hair to grow.

While herbal treatments are beneficial, they must be part of a broader approach that includes diet and stress management. Nutritional deficiencies and high stress levels can have a profound impact on hair health, leading to issues like hair thinning and loss. Ensuring a diet rich in proteins, omega-3 fatty acids, iron, and vitamins, especially Biotin (Vitamin B7) and Vitamin E, can significantly enhance hair growth and quality. Foods such as salmon, nuts, seeds, and green leafy vegetables are excellent sources of these nutrients. Moreover, managing stress through techniques like yoga, meditation, or regular exercise can reduce hair loss linked to stress and hormonal imbalances. By creating a balanced lifestyle that combines these practices with herbal remedies, you provide your hair with the best possible environment for growth and vitality, maintaining not just the health of your hair, but also enhancing your overall well-being. This holistic approach ensures that your efforts to nurture your hair are not just effective but also enriching to your life as a whole.

6.4 Anti-Aging Herbs for Skin Elasticity and Vitality

When exploring the realm of anti-aging, the focus often shifts towards maintaining skin elasticity and vitality, crucial markers of youthful, healthy skin. In this pursuit, the wisdom of herbal remedies offers not just a natural but a potent solution. Herbs like green tea and ginkgo biloba are celebrated not only for their health benefits but also for their significant antioxidant properties, which play a crucial role in supporting skin health. Green tea, rich in polyphenols such as catechins (a major group of flavonoids enriched in tea), offers profound anti-oxidant protection against free radical damage, which contributes to aging. These antioxidants help to maintain the integrity of the skin by slowing down the formation of fine lines and wrinkles. Ginkgo biloba, another powerhouse, contains flavonoids and terpenoids, compounds known for their strong antioxidant and anti-inflammatory properties. By enhancing blood circulation and increasing skin moisture retention, ginkgo biloba aids in maintaining the skin's elasticity and overall appearance, making it look more supple and vibrant.

Creating your own anti-aging serums and creams allows you to harness these botanical benefits directly. For a simple, effective serum, you can start with a green tea base. Brew a strong infusion of green tea, let it cool, then mix with aloe vera gel for its soothing properties and Vitamin E oil for added antioxidant power and skin repair benefits. This serum can be applied nightly under your moisturizer to help combat the daily oxidative stress your skin faces. For a more nourishing cream, incorporate ginkgo biloba extract, available at health stores, into a base of shea butter and jojoba oil. These carriers provide deep moisturization while the ginkgo extract works to protect and rejuvenate the skin cells. Apply this cream in the morning to shield your skin from environmental stressors throughout the day.

In addition to topical treatments, considering herbal supplements can significantly boost your skin health from the inside out. Supplements like green tea extract can provide a concentrated dose of its beneficial antioxidants without having to drink multiple cups of tea a day. Similarly, ginkgo biloba supplements can enhance circulatory health, which in turn supports the delivery of nutrients and oxygen to the skin, vital for its regeneration and repair. When selecting supplements, it's crucial to opt for those with high-quality, standardized extracts to ensure you receive the most potent benefits. Regular intake of these supplements, combined with a balanced diet rich in fruits, vegetables, and healthy fats, forms a robust foundation for maintaining youthful skin.

Protecting your skin from the sun and ensuring it remains hydrated are also fundamental components of an effective anti-aging skincare regimen. Sun exposure is one of the leading causes of premature aging, making sun protection essential. Opt for a mineral-based sunscreen that offers broad-spectrum protection without the harsh chemicals found in conventional sunscreens.

Reapply every two hours or immediately after swimming or sweating to maintain effective protection. Hydration, both internal and external, is equally crucial. Ensure you drink plenty of water throughout the day to maintain optimal hydration levels, which help keep your skin plump and elastic. Additionally, using hydrating sprays or setting your makeup with a mist infused with green tea can provide an extra hydration boost and add a protective layer against environmental pollutants.

By integrating these practices into your daily skincare routine, you actively contribute to preserving your skin's elasticity and vitality. This holistic approach not only combats the visible signs of aging but also enhances your skin's overall health, ensuring it remains resilient against the natural aging process. Through the meticulous selection of herbs, the creation of personalized skincare products, and the strategic use of supplements, you equip yourself with the tools necessary for maintaining youthful, radiant skin. This commitment not only beautifies but also strengthens your skin, reflecting your inner health and vitality in every glance in the mirror.

6.5 Soothing Herbal Remedies for Sunburn

When the skin has been overexposed to the sun's rays, it often retaliates with the painful redness and inflammation known as sunburn. While prevention is always preferable, there are times when the sun's embrace becomes too intense, and your skin pays the price. In such instances, the naturally soothing and cooling properties of aloe vera and lavender can provide much-needed relief. Aloe vera, renowned for its healing and anti-inflammatory properties, acts as a restorative balm for damaged skin. Its gel, which can be extracted directly from the plant leaf, forms a protective barrier that not only shields the skin from infection but also accelerates the healing process by improving blood circulation and reducing inflammation. Lavender, in addition to its calming scent, offers antiseptic and also anti-inflammatory properties that can soothe the pain of sunburn, reduce swelling, and facilitate the healing process. Applying a blend of aloe vera gel with a few drops of lavender essential oil can significantly cool the burn and aid in skin recovery. Note: If the skin is broken or blistered, please exercise caution and double check that you are not allergic to any ingredients used. Hydration plays a dual role in recovering from sunburn. Internally, drinking plenty of water is crucial after a sunburn as it helps the body replenish the fluids lost from sun exposure and heat. Externally, maintaining the skin's hydration is vital to the healing process. Cucumber, with its high water content and cooling properties, serves as an excellent hydrating agent for sunburned skin. It provides a soothing effect while delivering antioxidants that help manage the oxidative stress caused by UV rays. Blending cucumber into a pulp and applying it directly to sunburned areas not only soothes and cools the skin but also delivers moisture directly to the affected cells, promoting faster healing.

Creating your own DIY soothing gels and lotions allows for a personalized approach to treating sunburn, ensuring your skin receives optimal care with ingredients that are both effective and gentle. To create a soothing gel, start with pure aloe vera gel as a base, mix in cucumber juice for extra hydration, and add a few drops of lavender essential oil for its soothing properties. For a more comprehensive lotion, which can be used to treat larger areas of sunburn, mix aloe vera gel with a carrier oil like coconut or almond oil, which are known for their skin-healing fats. Add lavender and peppermint essential oils not only for their soothing effects but also for their very pleasant cooling sensation. Store this mixture in a cool place and apply generously to affected areas. The combination of these ingredients helps in reducing discomfort and accelerating the healing process, making the aftermath of a sunburn more bearable.

Sunburn prevention is far more manageable than treatment. While the soothing properties of herbs can aid in recovery, integrating preventive measures into your sun exposure routine can significantly reduce the risk of sunburn. Using natural, herbal-infused sunscreens provides a chemical-free option to protect your skin from UV rays.

Ingredients like zinc oxide or titanium dioxide can be mixed with oils like coconut and almond, which have natural SPF properties, to create a protective barrier on the skin. Wearing protective clothing, such as long-sleeved shirts, pants, and wide-brimmed hats, can also shield your skin from excessive sun exposure. Additionally, timing your sun exposure to avoid the peak hours between 10am and 4pm when the sun's rays are strongest can help minimize the risk of sunburn. Together, these strategies form a comprehensive approach to enjoying the sun safely, ensuring that your time outdoors is both enjoyable and kind to your skin.

6.6 Herbal Infusions for Bath and Body Care

The art of incorporating herbal infusions into your bath and body care routine transforms everyday rituals into sessions of rejuvenation and self-care. Focusing on the soothing properties of herbs like lavender and chamomile, you can create bath infusions that turn a simple soak into a therapeutic experience. Lavender, known for its calming and relaxing properties, works beautifully in a bath setting to alleviate stress and promote a restful night's sleep. Chamomile, with its mild sedative effects, complements lavender by soothing irritated skin and enhancing your ability to unwind. To prepare a bath infusion, fill a small cloth bag with dried lavender and chamomile flowers. Secure it tightly and let it steep in the bathwater as it fills.

The warm water will release the healing properties of the herbs, enveloping you in a fragrant, calming herbal embrace that eases the mind and pampers the skin.

Transitioning from relaxing baths to daily skincare, the preparation of herbal-infused oils offers a way to continuously nourish and moisturize the skin. Creating your own herbal oils is not only simple but allows you to tailor ingredients to your skin's needs. Start with a base oil like sweet almond or jojoba, which are excellent for most skin types due to their light texture and high nourishing properties. Infuse this oil with herbs such as calendula and rosemary, which promote healing and improve circulation, respectively. To infuse, gently heat the oil and add dried herbs, letting the mixture simmer on low heat for a few hours, ensuring the heat is not high enough to fry the herbs. Once done, strain the oil and store it in a dark glass bottle. Use this oil daily after bathing to lock in moisture and keep your skin supple and glowing.

The journey of herbal care extends to cleansing with natural body washes and soaps that gently purify without stripping the skin of its natural oils. Crafting your own soaps and washes allows you to incorporate herbs that cater specifically to your skin type while avoiding harsh chemicals. For a simple herbal body wash, start with a base of unscented castile soap, adding honey for its antibacterial properties and oatmeal for gentle exfoliation. Enhance this mixture with essential oils like tea tree for its antimicrobial properties and lavender for its soothing effect. This combination ensures that your skin is not only clean but also receives treatment for common issues like dryness and acne, maintaining healthy, vibrant skin.

Lastly, the soothing power of herbs can be particularly beneficial for tired, aching feet through herbal foot soaks. A foot soak with Epsom salts and herbs like peppermint and rosemary can relieve soreness and reduce inflammation. Peppermint provides a cooling sensation that soothes tired muscles, while rosemary enhances circulation, helping to rejuvenate overworked feet. Prepare this soak by dissolving Epsom salts in warm water and adding a few drops of peppermint and rosemary essential oils. Immersing your feet in this herbal concoction not only soothes and refreshes but also offers a moment of relaxation, grounding you after a long day.

As we wrap up this exploration into herbal infusions for bath and body care, it's clear that the integration of these natural elements into your routines not only enhances your physical well-being but also nurtures your mental and emotional health. Each herb selected and each product crafted carries with it the potential to transform ordinary routines into moments of wellness and tranquility. As you continue to explore and integrate these herbal practices, you foster a deeper connection with nature's rhythms, enhancing not just your beauty routines but also your overall quality of life.

Moving forward, the next chapter will delve into the vital world of immunity enhancement, exploring how herbs not only support but also fortify your body's natural defenses, continuing our journey towards holistic health and vibrant living.

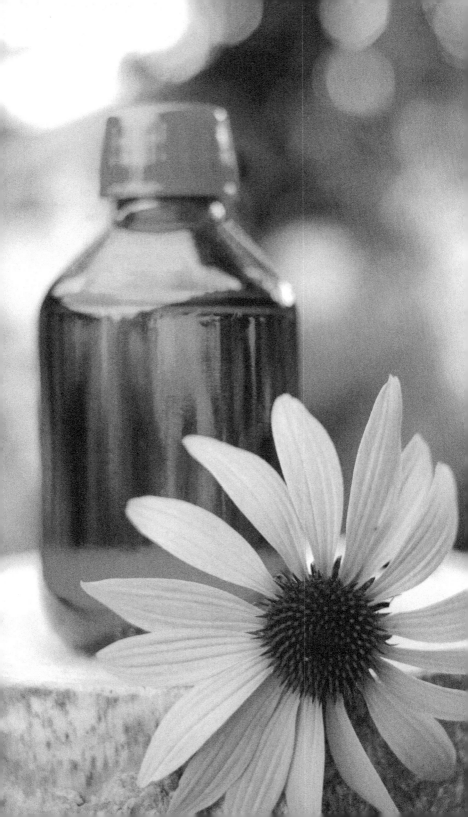

CHAPTER 7
IMMUNITY AND ENERGY BOOSTERS

As the seasons change, so too does the body's need for specific nutrients and support, particularly when it comes to our immune system. Amidst your busy life, you might often find yourself facing the double challenge of meeting professional deadlines and maintaining a robust immune system, especially during periods prone to colds and flu. This chapter is dedicated to uncovering the herbal allies that can bolster your immune defenses, seamlessly integrating them into your daily routine, and ensuring you remain energized and protected regardless of seasonal shifts.

7.1 Immune-Boosting Herbs for Seasonal Support

Imagine having natural guardians that stand ready to fortify your immune system at the first sign of a chill in the air. Echinacea, elderberry, and astragalus are not just herbs; they are your personal wellness warriors. Echinacea is renowned for its ability to enhance the immune response by increasing the production of white blood cells, which play a crucial role in fighting off infections. Its roots and leaves can be used to prepare teas and tinctures that help in shortening the duration of colds and flu. Elderberry is another powerhouse, packed with antioxidants and vitamins that boost your immune system. Its bioflavonoids and vitamins can help to reduce inflammation and lessen the severity of symptoms once a cold has taken hold. Astragalus, a staple in traditional Chinese medicine, is known for its deep immune-modulating effects. It supports and strengthens the immune system, promoting a general sense of well-being that is particularly useful during the colder months when the body is more susceptible to pathogens.

Creating an immune-supporting blend can be both a therapeutic and proactive measure against many seasonal illnesses. For a simple, effective tea, combine dried echinacea root, elderberry, and sliced astragalus root in equal parts. Steep this mixture in boiling water for about 15-20 minutes to make a potent herbal tea that can be consumed daily during flu season for immune support. For those on the go, tinctures can be a convenient option. Combine these herbs in a jar, cover them with alcohol and allow them to sit for a few weeks, shaking the mixture daily. Strain the liquid into a clean bottle, and use a dropper to take the tincture. This method extracts the active compounds efficiently, providing a concentrated dose that can be easily added to water or tea.

As the environment changes, so should your approach

to immune support. During the transitional periods from fall to winter and winter to spring, bolstering your immune system becomes essential. In addition to your herbal regimen, ensure that you get enough sunlight during the shorter days of fall and winter to maintain Vitamin D levels, which are vital for immune function. In the spring, when allergies can compromise your immune system, integrating stinging nettle into your diet can help mitigate allergic reactions and support overall immune health. This adaptability not only empowers you to maintain your health but also aligns your body's needs with the rhythms of nature.

Herbs are a powerful tool in the quest for health, but they work best when paired with a balanced diet and a healthy lifestyle. To support your immune system, focus on a diet rich in fruits, vegetables, lean proteins, and whole grains. These foods provide the necessary nutrients, such as Vitamins C and E, beta-carotene, and zinc, which are crucial for immune health. Regular physical activity, even something as simple as daily walking, can help boost your immune system by improving circulation and helping immune cells work more effectively. Sleep is another critical factor; ensuring you get 7-9 hours of quality sleep each night helps regenerate your body and strengthen your immune system.

To help you visualize the powerful alliance between

diet and herbal remedies, consider creating a chart that lists key immune-supporting foods alongside beneficial herbs. For instance, next to echinacea, note foods like citrus fruits rich in Vitamin C; pair elderberry with nuts and seeds that are high in Vitamin E; link astragalus with garlic and onions, which contain allicin, known for its immune-boosting properties. This visual guide can serve as a daily reminder of how you can fortify your body's defenses through integrated dietary and herbal strategies, ensuring that your immune system is as robust as your schedule demands.

7.2 Energizing Herbs to Combat Fatigue

In the relentless pursuit of balancing personal and professional life, feeling energetically depleted can often seem like an inevitable outcome. However, turning to the natural world reveals potent allies like ginseng, rhodiola, and maca, each distinguished not only by their ability to enhance vitality but also by their capacity to provide energy without the jittery side effects associated with caffeine. Ginseng, revered in traditional medicine for its energizing properties, works by improving the efficiency of energy production in your cells thanks to its bioactive compounds known as ginsenosides. This adaptogenic herb aids in fighting fatigue and enhances mental clarity, making it an invaluable resource for those demanding days. Rhodiola, another robust adaptogen, stimulates your body's stress-response system to increase energy production and reduce exhaustion. Its active ingredients, rosavin and salidroside, help elevate the capacity for mental work and endurance, particularly under stressful conditions. Maca, a root indigenous to the Andes, is traditionally used to boost stamina and endurance. It contains compounds known as macamides, which are unique to the plant and are thought to be directly responsible for its energy-boosting properties.

Integrating these herbs into your morning routine can transform the start of your day. Imagine beginning your day not just with a cup of coffee but with a revitalizing herbal tonic that not only wakes you up but also nourishes your body. Crafting a morning tonic can be simple and enjoyable. You might start with a teaspoon of maca powder and a small amount of rhodiola extract added to a smoothie. Blend this with fresh fruits for sweetness and a handful of spinach for an extra nutrient kick. For those who prefer a warm beverage, preparing a ginseng tea by steeping sliced ginseng root in hot water can be a comforting alternative. Adding a slice of lemon or a bit of honey can enhance the flavor and add to the invigorating properties of the tea. Consuming these tonics as part of your morning ritual sets a positive tone for the day, ensuring you are primed with natural, sustained energy.

Managing stress is crucial for maintaining high energy

levels throughout the day. Stress, particularly chronic stress, can deplete your energy reserves and leave you feeling exhausted. Adaptogenic herbs like rhodiola and ginseng support your body in balancing stress hormones such as cortisol, which, when elevated, can lead to fatigue. Incorporating these herbs into your daily regimen helps modulate your body's stress response, preserving your energy for more prolonged periods. This might involve taking a standardized extract of rhodiola in capsule form during breakfast or sipping ginseng tea mid-morning. By managing stress effectively with these herbs, you not only enhance your immediate energy levels but also contribute to long-term vitality.

Encouraging a balanced approach to rest and activity is essential for sustaining energy. While it may seem counter-intuitive, regular physical activity increases your energy levels and combats fatigue. Gentle activities like yoga or brisk walking can significantly boost your energy through improved blood flow and increased endorphin levels. Pairing this with adequate rest, which allows your body to recover and rejuvenate, is essential. Herbal aids like maca can be particularly beneficial here, as they provide the necessary energy boost without interfering with your body's natural sleep cycle. Adding a spoonful of maca powder to a post-workout shake can help replenish your energy reserves without compromising your night-time rest. This balanced approach ensures that you maintain optimal energy levels, supported by natural herbal remedies, allowing you to meet the demands of your day with vitality and enthusiasm.

7.3 Herbs for Cold and Flu Prevention

In the realm of natural health, being proactive is key, especially when it comes to combating the common cold and flu. This proactive approach not only involves lifestyle and dietary choices but also the strategic use of specific herbs that can prevent and alleviate these ailments. Garlic, ginger, and thyme stand out as natural defenders against respiratory infections, each bringing unique properties that support your body's ability to fend off illnesses.

Garlic has been celebrated for centuries not only for its robust flavor but also for its potent antimicrobial properties. It contains allicin, a compound that is released when garlic is crushed or chopped and is known for its ability to fight bacteria and viruses. Incorporating garlic into your diet can therefore act as a preventative measure during flu season. You might add freshly minced garlic to dishes like soups, sauces, and stir-fries, which not only enhances the flavor of your meals but also fortifies your immune system. For those who might find the taste too strong, aged garlic supplements are a more palatable alternative that retains the health benefits without the intense flavor.

Ginger, with its warm, spicy profile, is another powerful herb for preventing colds and flu. Its anti-inflammatory and anti-oxidant properties help to soothe the throat, reduce cough, and lower fever. A simple yet effective way to use ginger is to brew it into a tea. You can slice fresh ginger root, simmer it in hot water for about 20 minutes, and add a touch of honey and lemon for taste. This not only helps in preventing respiratory infections but also provides a comforting, warming beverage that can uplift your spirits on a cold day.

Thyme is often overshadowed in discussions about immune health, but its benefits are profound. Rich in thymol, an essential oil with natural antiseptic properties, Thyme is excellent for respiratory health. It can help alleviate coughs by relaxing the muscles of the trachea and reducing inflammation. A tea made from thyme leaves can be a simple yet effective remedy during cold and flu season. Steep dried thyme in hot water for about 10 minutes, strain, and sip. This herb's powerful effects can help clear your respiratory tract, making breathing easier and preventing infections from taking hold.

When the initial signs of a cold or flu emerge, acting swiftly with herbal remedies can significantly shorten the duration and severity of the illness. Elderberry syrup is a standout remedy, known for its antiviral properties and ability to boost immune response. At the first sign of illness, taking a tablespoon of elderberry syrup several times a day can help interfere with virus replication and speed up recovery. For sore throats, a gargle made from salt water and a few drops of eucalyptus oil can provide immediate relief. Eucalyptus has antimicrobial properties that can help reduce swelling and clear mucus. A warming tea made from a blend of yarrow, elderflower, and peppermint can also be beneficial at the onset of cold symptoms. Yarrow is known for its fever-reducing properties, elderflower helps clear congestion, and peppermint soothes the stomach and reduces headaches. Brew these herbs together to create a potent tea that not only fights the virus but also alleviates your symptoms, helping you feel better faster.

Maintaining respiratory health is crucial, especially during the colder months. Herbs like mullein and licorice root are beneficial for keeping the respiratory tract healthy and clear. Mullein in particular, is known for its soothing effect on the bronchioles. Its leaves and flowers can be used to prepare a tea that helps in expelling mucus and easing chest congestion. Licorice root, with its sweet, earthy flavor, has a soothing effect and acts as an expectorant, helping to loosen and expel mucus. A simple tea made from licorice root can be a comforting way to support lung health and prevent respiratory ailments.

To ensure you are always prepared at the first sign of a cold or flu, assembling a herbal cold and flu kit is a wise strategy. This kit should include echinacea tincture, known for its immune-boosting properties; elderberry syrup for its antiviral effects; a blend of dried yarrow, elderflower, and peppermint for making tea; and capsules of garlic and ginger for their antimicrobial benefits.

Additionally, include a small bottle of eucalyptus oil and a pack of licorice tea. Keep this kit in an easily accessible place at home, and consider preparing a smaller, portable version for your workplace or car. With these tools at your disposal, you can confidently manage the onset of cold and flu symptoms, supporting your body's natural defenses and ensuring a quicker return to health.

7.4 Natural Antibiotics: Herbal Powerhouses

In the quest for maintaining health and treating infections, the natural world offers potent solutions that have been utilized long before the advent of modern pharmaceuticals. Among these, herbs like oregano and goldenseal stand out for their remarkable antibacterial properties. Oregano, a common culinary herb, is imbued with compounds such as carvacrol and thymol, which have been shown to possess strong antibacterial and antifungal activities. These compounds work by disrupting the pathogen cell membrane, effectively neutralizing harmful bacteria without promoting antibiotic resistance. Goldenseal, often used in traditional medicine, contains berberine, a compound known for its broad-spectrum antibiotic properties. Berberine fights bacterial infection by inhibiting bacteria's ability to attach to human cells, which is crucial in preventing and treating infections, particularly those of the mucous membranes.

Creating effective herbal antibiotic formulas requires more than just knowledge of which herbs have antibacterial properties; it involves understanding how to synergistically combine these herbs to enhance their efficacy. One potent herbal antibiotic blend can be created by combining tinctures of oregano, goldenseal, and echinacea. While oregano provides robust antibacterial action, goldenseal serves as a mucous membrane tonic, and echinacea enhances overall immune function, creating a comprehensive defense strategy against bacterial infections. To prepare this blend, mix equal parts of each herb's tincture in a dark glass dropper bottle.

This formula can be administered by adding a few drops to water or juice at the onset of an infection, providing a powerful, natural means to enhance the body's ability to fight off bacterial pathogens.

Understanding when to use these herbal antibiotics is crucial for their effective application. These natural remedies are best utilized at the onset of symptoms indicative of bacterial infections, such as unusual mucous production, skin inflammation, or digestive disturbances.

However, it's important to recognize the limitations of herbal treatments and know when to seek conventional medical advice. Severe infections, such as those that are rapidly progressing, involve high fevers, or are potentially life-threatening, should be evaluated by a healthcare professional. In such cases, conventional antibiotics may be necessary to effectively treat the infection and prevent complications.

Maintaining gut health is paramount when using herbs with antibiotic properties, as the disruption of the body's natural bacterial flora can sometimes lead to digestive imbalances. Both oregano and goldenseal, while effective against harmful bacteria, can also affect beneficial gut bacteria if used indiscriminately. To mitigate this, it's advisable to pair these herbal antibiotics with probiotics, which can help maintain a healthy balance of gut flora. Taking a high-quality probiotic supplement several hours apart from the herbal antibiotic ensures that the probiotic bacteria are not immediately neutralized by the antibacterial herbs, allowing them to colonize the gut effectively. Additionally, incorporating fermented foods such as yogurt, kefir, and sauerkraut into your diet can further support gut health by providing a natural source of probiotics.

Incorporating these practices into your approach to treating infections allows you to harness the powerful anti-bacterial properties of herbs like oregano and goldenseal, while also ensuring the health of your digestive system and overall well-being. By understanding the appropriate use and potential impacts of these herbal remedies, you empower yourself with natural solutions that support your body's health in a balanced and effective way. This approach not only aligns with a holistic view of health care but also respects the complexity of the human body and the intricacies of its interactions with the natural world.

7.5 Adaptogenic Herbs for Long-Term Energy

Adaptogens, a select group of herbs including ashwagandha and holy basil, have gained recognition for their unique ability to enhance stamina and manage stress, which are crucial for maintaining long-term energy. Unlike stimulants that produce a quick surge of energy followed by a crash, adaptogens support sustained energy levels by modulating the adrenal system. Ashwagandha, for instance, works by normalizing the levels of cortisol, the stress hormone, in the body. Elevated cortisol can lead to adrenal fatigue, which is often manifested by a chronic feeling of tiredness. By regulating cortisol levels, ashwagandha helps maintain consistent energy throughout the day. Holy basil operates on a similar premise but also enhances the body's efficient use of oxygen, which is vital for energy production. These herbs do not just temporarily relieve fatigue; they help the body adapt to stress and exertion, enhancing overall vitality and stamina.

Incorporating these adaptogens into your daily life can be both simple and transformative. For continuous energy and stress management, you might start your day with a cup of ashwagandha tea. This can be prepared by simmering a teaspoon of the powdered root in water for about 15 minutes; adding cinnamon and honey can enhance the flavor and also provide additional blood sugar stabilization, which further aids in maintaining energy levels. Alternatively, holy basil leaves can be used to brew a refreshing tea, perfect for afternoon slumps; just steep the leaves in hot water as you would with any herbal tea and enjoy the uplifting effects. Another practical way to include these adaptogens in your routine is through the use of capsules or tinctures, which are convenient and can be easily integrated into your morning or evening health regimen, ensuring you do not miss out on their benefits even on your busiest days.

The impact of adaptogens extends beyond daily energy enhancement to improving athletic performance and recovery. For athletes or anyone engaged in regular physical activity, maintaining energy levels and recovering quickly from workouts is vital. Adaptogens like rhodiola are particularly known for their ability to increase endurance and reduce recovery time. Its active components help increase the synthesis of ATP, the primary energy molecule in the body, which is crucial during physical activities. Incorporating rhodiola, either in capsule form or as a tea, about an hour before exercise can provide the stamina needed for a more intense and prolonged workout. Post-exercise, adaptogens such as ashwagandha can be invaluable in reducing muscle fatigue and speeding up recovery by mitigating the oxidative stress that occurs during strenuous activities.

Personalizing the use of adaptogens to fit individual needs and circumstances is crucial for maximizing their benefits. The key to effective use lies in understanding your body's responses and adjusting accordingly. If you are new to adaptogens, starting with low doses and gradually increasing as your body adapts is advisable. Monitoring how you feel daily can provide insights into how well an adaptogen is working for you. For instance, if you notice an improvement in your energy levels or a reduction in stress symptoms with regular use of holy basil, you might decide to make it a staple in your stress management toolkit. On the other hand, if you are an athlete looking to enhance recovery, experimenting with rhodiola and noting changes in your post-workout recovery could guide whether it should be a regular part of your regimen. Since adaptogens work best when used consistently, finding those that you can easily incorporate into your daily routine, and that you respond well to, will help you achieve the best results. This personalized approach ensures that you are not only adopting a natural solution but also one that is harmoniously aligned with your body's unique needs and your lifestyle, enhancing your overall vitality and capacity to handle the demands of your day.

7.6 Vitamin and Mineral-Rich Herbs for Overall Health

In the pursuit of optimal health, the role of vitamins and minerals cannot be overstated, and nature offers a bounty of nutrient-dense herbs that can significantly contribute to our nutritional intake. Among these, spirulina and chlorella stand out as superfoods due to their remarkable concentration of nutrients. Spirulina, a type of blue-green algae, is celebrated for its high protein content, which includes all essential amino acids, making it an excellent supplement for vegetarians and vegans. It is also rich in B-vitamins, iron, and manganese, which play crucial roles in energy metabolism and antioxidant protection. Chlorella, another algae, is highly regarded for its detoxifying properties and its impressive array of vitamins, including Vitamin C, and minerals such as magnesium and zinc, essential for immune function and overall cellular health.

The debate between choosing herbal supplements versus consuming whole food herbs is piercing in the context of these nutrient powerhouses. While supplements can provide concentrated doses of specific nutrients, whole food forms of herbs like spirulina and chlorella offer a complex matrix of nutrients that work synergistically. This complexity not only aids in the more natural absorption of these nutrients by the body but also ensures that you benefit from additional phytonutrients ("Phyto" refers to the Greek word for plant. These chemicals help protect plants from germs, fungi, bugs, and other threats) that are often absent in isolated supplements. For instance, the fibrous cell walls of chlorella bind with heavy metals and toxins in the digestive tract, aiding in their removal and providing a cleanse that isolated supplements might not offer.

Integrating these nutritious herbs into your daily diet can be both simple and transformative. Spirulina can be easily added to smoothies, providing a nutrient boost without significantly altering the taste of your favorite blends. Its vibrant green color can also add visual appeal to foods like salads or dressings, where it can be sprinkled in powder form. Chlorella tablets are another convenient way to incorporate this herb into your routine, especially for those who are frequently on-the-go. For those who enjoy culinary experimentation, chlorella can be used in baking or as a garnish on soups and stews, where it can add a subtle flavor and a boost of nutrients.

The impact of including these vitamin and mineral-rich herbs in your diet extends beyond just meeting your nutritional needs; it supports your overall physical and mental well-being. The dense nutrient profile of spirulina and chlorella supports immune function, aids in detoxification, and can improve energy levels, making them a valuable addition to any diet. Moreover, the antioxidants present in these herbs help combat oxidative stress, a common culprit in aging and many chronic diseases. By reducing oxidative stress, these herbs not only contribute to long-term health but also improve your day-to-day functioning, helping you feel more vibrant and energetic.

Incorporating spirulina and chlorella into your diet doesn't just nourish your body; it aligns you with a holistic approach to health that emphasizes the power of natural foods to heal and sustain us. As you continue to explore the vast world of herbal remedies, remember that each small step you take in integrating these powerful plants into your life not only enhances your health but also deepens your connection to the natural world. This chapter has opened up avenues to strengthen your body's defenses and invigorate your spirit, paving the way for a deeper exploration of natural healing modalities in the upcoming chapters, where we will delve into the rejuvenating world of natural skincare and beauty enhancements. This journey into the healing powers of herbs is not just about enhancing health but about transforming lifestyles and enriching experiences, ensuring that every aspect of your well-being is nurtured and cherished.

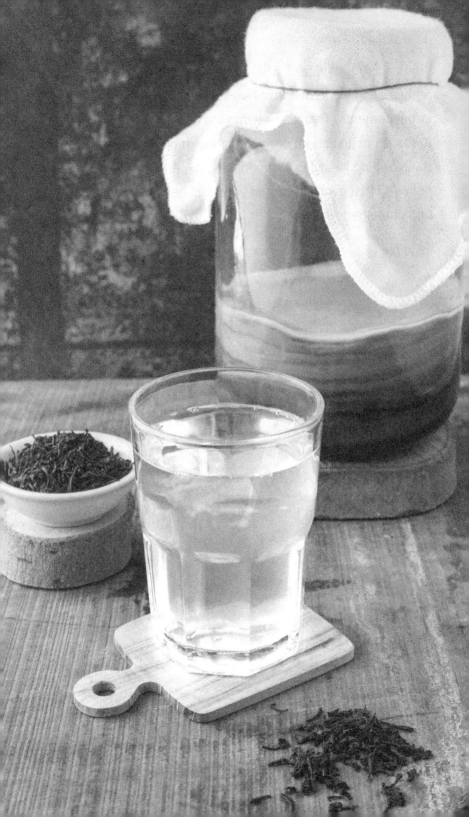

CHAPTER 8
ADVANCED APPLICATIONS AND PRACTICES

In the verdant embrace of your own garden lies the potential for profound healing and wellness. Cultivating your personal collection of medicinal herbs is not merely about adding beauty to your environment; it's about enriching your life with plants that offer therapeutic benefits right at your fingertips. This chapter guides you through the gratifying process of growing, harvesting, and utilizing your own herbs, transforming your garden into a sanctuary of health and healing.

8.1 Growing Your Own Medicinal Herbs

Choosing the right herbs for your garden requires consideration of your local climate and the space available. Whether you have sprawling yard space or a modest balcony for containers, there's an array of herbs suited to your growing conditions. Start by researching which herbs thrive naturally in your area. For instance, lavender and rosemary adore the warm, dry conditions of the Mediterranean, while cilantro and parsley might prefer the cooler, milder temperatures. Utilize local planting guides or consult with a nursery expert to select herbs that will not only grow well but will also meet your specific health needs. For beginners, easy-to-grow herbs like mint, lemon balm, and basil can be particularly rewarding, as they are both hardy and versatile in their uses.

Setting the foundation for a thriving herb garden begins with understanding the basics of soil preparation, planting, and maintenance. Most medicinal herbs favor well-draining soil as waterlogged roots can lead to plant diseases. Enhancing your garden soil with organic matter like compost not only improves drainage but also enriches the soil with nutrients. When planting, give each herb ample space to expand - crowded plants compete for resources and are more prone to illness. Regular maintenance involves watering, weeding, and pruning to encourage healthy growth. Additionally, some herbs, such as mint, can be invasive; these should be contained in pots to prevent them from overtaking your garden.

Harvesting your herbs at the right time is crucial for maximizing their medicinal properties. Generally, the best time to harvest is just before the plants bloom, as this is when their oils and flavors are most potent. Harvest in the morning after the dew has dried but before the sun is at its peak, to ensure the essential oils are concentrated.

Drying is the most common method for preserving herbs and can be done using a food dehydrator, an oven on a low setting, or naturally air-dried in a warm, dry place. Store dried herbs in airtight containers away from light and heat to maintain their potency.

Transforming your home-grown herbs into medicinal preparations like tinctures, teas, and salves allows you to personalize your health remedies and ensures you're using the freshest, most potent botanicals. For instance, creating a calming tea blend is as simple as drying lavender and chamomile, which can be steeped in hot water to soothe stress. Salves made from calendula and comfrey can be used to heal skin irritations and minor wounds. Tinctures, which are concentrated herbal extracts made using alcohol, can be prepared from herbs like echinacea or valerian to boost immune function or aid sleep.

To aid in your planning and planting, consider creating a herb compatibility chart. This visual guide can help you determine which herbs grow well together and which should be planted apart. For example, rosemary and sage thrive in similar dry conditions and can be planted close to each other, while mint should be kept in separate containers to avoid overtaking neighboring plants. This chart serves as a handy reference when designing your garden layout, ensuring each herb has the best possible conditions for growth, ultimately leading to a more bountiful harvest.

In cultivating your own medicinal garden, you not only gain access to fresh herbs but also deepen your connection with the natural world. Each plant you nurture and each remedy you create from your garden carries the essence of care, personalized to support your specific health needs. As you watch your garden thrive, you'll find that these plants do more than just grow - they become a living, breathing extension of your health and well-being, rooted in the very soil of your home.

8.2 Herbal Fermentation: Kombucha and Beyond

The craft of fermentation, a practice as ancient as any, brings with it a host of benefits that extend far beyond simple preservation. Today, herbal fermentation stands as a bridge connecting traditional wisdom with modern health practices, offering unique ways to enhance both the flavor and nutritional profile of everyday herbs. At the heart of this practice lies the ability to harness beneficial bacteria and yeasts to convert simple sugars into ethanol and acids, thereby imbuing the herbs with a complexity that boosts their health benefits significantly. These probiotic-rich concoctions not only improve digestion and enhance the bioavailability of nutrients but will also strengthen the immune system.

Kombucha, a fizzy tea-based beverage, has soared in popularity as a staple of herbal fermentation. To start your own kombucha, you'll need a SCOBY (Symbiotic Culture Of Bacteria and Yeast), which acts as the fermenting powerhouse, transforming sweetened tea into a nutrient-rich elixir. Begin by preparing a base tea - green or black works beautifully - infused with your choice of medicinal herbs. Chamomile or lavender can add calming properties, while ginger boosts its digestive benefits. Once the tea is steeped and sweetened with sugar, cool it to room temperature before adding the SCOBY. Cover the concoction with a breathable cloth to prevent contaminants while allowing air to circulate. Over the course of 7-14 days, the SCOBY will metabolize the sugar, and the tea will start to ferment, developing layers of flavor and increasing in probiotic content. The final product, a tangy and effervescent drink, can be consumed daily to reap its digestive and energetic benefits.

Expanding beyond kombucha, the realm of herbal fermentation offers myriad possibilities for creative and healthful projects. Kefir, a fermented milk drink, can be crafted with a water-based variant to incorporate herbal infusions. Try adding rose petals or hibiscus to water kefir grains for a drink that's not only visually stunning but also heart-supportive and rich in antioxidants. Herbal beers, another ancient tradition, allow for the brewing of low alcohol options that are brimming with the flavors and benefits of herbs like stinging nettle or dandelion - both known for their detoxifying properties. Fermented herbal pastes, made from herbs like garlic, turmeric, and horse-radish, can be used as condiments that boost both the nutrient content and flavor profile of meals.

When fermenting herbs at home, safety and proper storage are paramount to ensure that your creations are both delicious and beneficial. Always use clean, sterilized equipment to avoid introducing harmful bacteria into your ferments. Glass jars are preferable as they do not react with the acids produced during fermentation. Keep your ferments in a cool, dark place to maintain the activity of beneficial bacteria without over-fermenting the product. Once ready, transferring your ferments to the refrigerator will slow down the fermentation process and preserve their flavors and nutritional benefits longer. Always check for signs of mold or unpleasant odors; these can indicate contamination and should be discarded immediately.

By integrating the art of herbal fermentation into your well-ness routine, you not only connect with ancient traditions but also contribute to your health in dynamic ways. Each sip of kombucha or bite of a fermented paste connects you to a cycle of wellness that is supported by the very microbes that thrive within these preparations. This process, deeply rooted in the natural world, exemplifies how traditional practices can be revitalized to fit modern needs, enriching our lives with flavors and health benefits that are as old as time.

8.3 Herbal First Aid Kit: Common Ailments

In the realm of natural healing, having a well-prepared herbal first aid kit is akin to holding a treasury of remedies that can swiftly address common ailments - from the sudden scrape to an unexpected stomach upset. Imagine the peace of mind that comes from knowing you possess the tools to soothe a burn, calm an insect sting, or alleviate indigestion, all with substances derived from nature and crafted by your own hands. This section not only outlines essential herbal remedies to include in your first aid arsenal but also provides detailed guidance on how to prepare and effectively use these remedies, ensuring you're ready to handle minor emergencies with confidence and care.

Your herbal first aid kit should be versatile and comprehensive, addressing a range of common issues that you and your family may encounter. Key items include aloe vera gel, known for its soothing properties on burns and skin irritations; calendula salve, which can be applied to cuts and scrapes for its wound-healing benefits; lavender oil, a multipurpose essential oil that alleviates stress, disinfects wounds, and reduces pain; and peppermint oil, excellent for its anti-nausea effects and soothing relief on itchy insect bites. Additionally, keeping a small supply of activated charcoal can be invaluable for its ability to absorb toxins, making it a go-to remedy for digestive disturbances caused by food poisoning.

Preparing your own herbal remedies ensures that you know exactly what goes into each product, allowing you to tailor them to your specific health needs and preferences. To start, a simple calendula salve can be made by infusing olive oil with dried calendula flowers for several weeks in a cool, dark place. Strain the flowers out, and gently heat the infused oil with beeswax until the wax melts. Pour this mixture into small tins or jars to cool; you now have a healing salve that can be applied to bruises, cuts, and rashes. For a quick and effective tincture, echinacea can be steeped in vodka or another high-proof alcohol, which extracts its antimicrobial properties - ideal for cleansing wounds or boosting the immune system at the onset of a cold.

Understanding when and how to use each item in your herbal first aid kit maximizes their effectiveness. Aloe vera gel should be applied directly to burns or sunburns to soothe and promote healing. For insect bites, a drop of peppermint oil can provide immediate relief from itching and swelling. If you experience indigestion or nausea, sipping a tea made from peppermint or ginger can be soothing. In instances of cuts or scrapes, clean the area thoroughly with water or a mild soap before applying calendula salve to the affected area to enhance healing. Always remember that while these remedies are effective for minor ailments, more serious or persistent conditions require professional medical attention.

Sharing your knowledge of herbal first aid not only enhances the self-sufficiency of your community but also deepens your own understanding and appreciation for herbal medicine. Consider organizing small workshops with friends or family where you can demonstrate how to prepare basic herbal remedies. Create simple hand-outs that outline what each herb in your first aid kit can be used for, and perhaps even prepare small kits that your attendees can take home. In doing so, you foster a community that values and understands the importance of natural healing, equipping those you care about with the skills to treat everyday ailments with confidence and natural efficacy.

By crafting and utilizing your own herbal first aid kit, you embrace the role of both healer and teacher, passing on traditional wisdom that has supported human health for generations. As you blend, concoct, and apply these natural remedies, you become more attuned to the needs of your body and more connected to the natural world, ensuring that you and your loved ones are cared for with nature's own provisions.

8.4 Crafting Herbal Gifts: Ideas for Every Occasion

Creating and giving herbal gifts is a heartfelt way to share the beauty and benefits of nature with friends and loved ones. Whether for a birthday, a holiday, or just to show appreciation, gifts made from herbs offer a personal touch that can be both soothing and healing. Picture a beautifully wrapped package containing homemade herbal soaps, a jar of infused oil, or a collection of calming tea blends - these are gifts that not only please the senses but also provide wellness benefits that store-bought items rarely offer.

When considering what herbal gifts to make, think about the preferences and needs of the person receiving them. For someone who loves cooking, an array of infused oils can be a delightful surprise. You can create these by gently heating olive oil with herbs like rosemary, thyme, or basil. Once the oil captures the essence of the herbs, strain it and pour it into elegant bottles. Add a tag describing each infusion's ideal culinary uses. For tea lovers, assemble a selection of herbal tea blends using dried herbs such as chamomile for relaxation, peppermint for digestion, or lavender for a soothing nighttime brew. Place the teas in a decorative box or tin, complete with labels and brewing instructions. If your recipient enjoys pampering themselves, consider crafting bath salts or soaps using herbs like lavender or calendula, known for their soothing and skin-healing properties. Bath salts can be made by mixing Epsom salts with dried lavender flowers and a few drops of essential oil, providing a spa-like experience at home.

Presentation is key when it comes to herbal gifts, as it enhances the overall experience and shows the thought put into the gift. Opt for natural and sustainable packaging materials to reflect the eco-friendly nature of herbal products. Use glass jars, metal tins, or cloth bags that can be reused or recycled. Decorate with natural twine, dried flowers, or handwritten tags to add a personal touch. For soaps, use brown paper or linen cloth for wrapping, and seal them with a wax stamp for a vintage feel. When packaging liquids like infused oils, ensure the containers are sealed properly to prevent leaks and choose bottles that are both aesthetically pleasing and functional. Adding a custom label with the recipient's name or a thoughtful message can turn a simple bottle of herb-infused oil into a cherished keep-sake.

Including instructions and a detailed description of the benefits of each herbal gift is not only thoughtful but also increases the value of the gift. People appreciate knowing not just what they are receiving but also how it can benefit them. For each item in the herbal gift basket, include a small card or booklet that details how to use the product, the benefits of the included herbs, and any necessary precautions. For example, if you're giving a sleep-promoting tea blend, include a note explaining how the herbs help with relaxation and the best time to consume the tea for optimal benefits. This not only educates them, but also enhances their experience, making the herbal gift more meaningful and appreciated.

By taking the time to craft personalized herbal gifts, you not only provide something unique and thoughtful but also promote a healthier, more natural lifestyle. Each gift becomes a reflection of your care and commitment to wellbeing, wrapped in a package that delights and heals. This approach to gifting not only strengthens personal connections but also extends the healing power of herbs beyond your own home, spreading wellness and the joys of herbal remedies to those around you.

8.5 Ancient Herbal Traditions Meets Modern Science

In an era where high-tech health innovations are celebrated, there's profound wisdom in pausing and reflecting on the ancient paths of herbal medicine. These traditions, honed over millennia, are not just historical footnotes but are vibrant, living practices that offer tangible health benefits, validated increasingly by modern scientific research. The integration of these age-old herbal practices with contemporary scientific methods not only enriches our understanding but also enhances the efficacy and application of herbal medicine today. This synergy invites a balanced perspective where respect for tradition complements the rigor of science, creating a holistic approach to health that honors the past while embracing the future.

One striking example of ancient remedies gaining scientific endorsement is the use of turmeric, known for its anti-inflammatory properties. Traditionally used in Ayurvedic medicine to treat a plethora of ailments from arthritis to digestive disorders, turmeric's active component, curcumin, has been extensively studied in the West for its potent anti-inflammatory and antioxidant properties. Research has shown that curcumin can match and sometimes surpass the effectiveness of some anti-inflammatory drugs, without the side effects, offering a natural alternative for managing inflammation and pain. Gingko biloba, used for centuries in Chinese medicine to enhance cognitive function, has been the subject of numerous clinical trials that support its efficacy in improving blood circulation and promoting brain health, particularly in geriatric patients.

The knowledge of traditional herbalists, often passed down through generations, provides invaluable insights into the holistic use of plants that goes beyond their biochemical components. For instance, traditional healers often approach remedies in the context of the individual's overall environment and lifestyle, a practice that modern medicine is beginning to appreciate under the banner of personalized medicine. Learning from these herbalists, modern practitioners can adopt a more integrative approach to health, viewing the individual as a whole rather than a set of symptoms to be treated in isolation. This holistic approach not only enhances the therapeutic relationship but also improves the effectiveness of the treatment by tailoring it to the individual's unique context.

Looking ahead, the future of herbal medicine appears vibrant, promising a richer integration of scientific validation and ancient wisdom. As more research is focused on herbal medicine, spurred by growing public interest and the limitations of conventional drugs, we are likely to see a deeper scientific understanding of the mechanisms behind herbal remedies. This could lead to more precise dosages, better safety profiles, and enhanced efficacy of herbal treatments. Moreover, with the rising interest in sustainability and natural products, herbal medicine stands poised to become a more prominent player in global health practices. It offers a pathway to healing that is not only effective but also aligns with the principles of ecological sustainability and personal well-being.

The convergence of ancient herbal traditions and modern

science is not just a testament to the enduring power of these practices but also a call to foster a deeper, more respectful partnership between different ways of knowing. It challenges us to think globally and act locally, to blend the wisdom of the old with the innovations of the new in our quest for health and healing. As we continue to explore and validate the rich tapestry of herbal medicine, we weave a new narrative of health care - one that is as dynamic and complex as the natural world from which these remedies arise.

8.6 Setting Up Your Home Apothecary for Success

Creating a home apothecary is akin to designing a personal wellness sanctuary - a space where the healing powers of nature are within arm's reach. When you decide to establish this dedicated area in your home, you're committing to a lifestyle that values self-care and natural living. The design of your apothecary should reflect both functionality and your personal aesthetic, making it a welcoming and efficient space where you can prepare and store your herbal remedies.

To design your home apothecary, consider the specific conditions that herbs need to maintain their potency - cool, dark, and dry. Choose a space away from direct sunlight, perhaps a pantry, a cabinet in a quiet corner of your kitchen, or a designated room if space allows.

Wooden shelves or glass-fronted cabinets are not just practical for organizing jars and containers but also add a touch of rustic charm. Ensure that each shelf is tall enough to accommodate bottles of varying sizes, from small tincture bottles to larger jars for bulk dried herbs. Labeling each jar clearly with the herb's name, date of acquisition or harvest, and any special storage instructions is crucial for easy navigation and effective use. For an added touch of personal style, use uniform jars with custom labels that reflect your home's decor, creating a cohesive look that is both beautiful and practical.

Stocking your apothecary involves more than just filling shelves with herbs. Start by selecting a range of herbs that target your specific health needs - calming herbs like lavender and chamomile if stress is a frequent concern, or digestive aids like peppermint and ginger. Essential tools such as mortar and pestle for grinding herbs, a scale for precise measurement, and various sizes of sieves are also critical for preparing your remedies.

Additionally, stock carrier oils like almond and jojoba, beeswax for salves, alcohol for tinctures, and a variety of tea infusers and strainers. Investing in high-quality, organic herbs is essential, as is ensuring you have a good mix of forms, including powders, dried leaves, and flowers, to suit different types of preparations.

Maintaining your apothecary is crucial to ensure that your herbs and preparations remain potent and safe to use. Regularly check your stock for any signs of spoilage or pest infestation, which can occur even with the best storage conditions. Herbs generally have a shelf life of one to three years, depending on the herb and storage conditions; any herbs that have lost their color, scent, or flavor should be composted and replaced. Clean your containers and tools regularly to avoid cross-contamination and maintain the efficacy of your herbal remedies. This maintenance not only ensures your preparations are effective but also deepens your relationship with the tools and ingredients you use, fostering a greater appreciation and understanding of the herbal preparation process.

Ethical and sustainable practices are the cornerstone of a truly holistic home apothecary. This encompasses not only how you source your herbs - opting for suppliers who prioritize sustainable and ethical harvesting practices - but also how you manage waste in your apothecary. Implement practices such as composting spent herbs and reusing or recycling jars and bottles. When possible, grow your own herbs, which not only reduces your carbon footprint but also enhances your connection to the healing plants you use. Engaging with local herbalists and participating in community exchanges can also enrich your practice and ensure it supports, each step - from designing the space to choosing and caring for your herbs - reflects a commitment to living a life in harmony with nature. This space becomes a physical manifestation of your health ideals, a daily reminder of your dedication to nurturing yourself and your loved ones with the gifts of the earth. As you blend, brew, and concoct, your apothecary is not just a collection of shelves and jars but a vibrant, living archive of nature's bounty, tailored to heal, soothe, and rejuvenate.

As you close this chapter on setting up your home apothecary, the knowledge and insights gained here seamlessly weave into the broader tapestry of natural wellness explored throughout this book. Each chapter builds upon the last, guiding you deeper into understanding and utilizing the vast potential of herbal medicine.

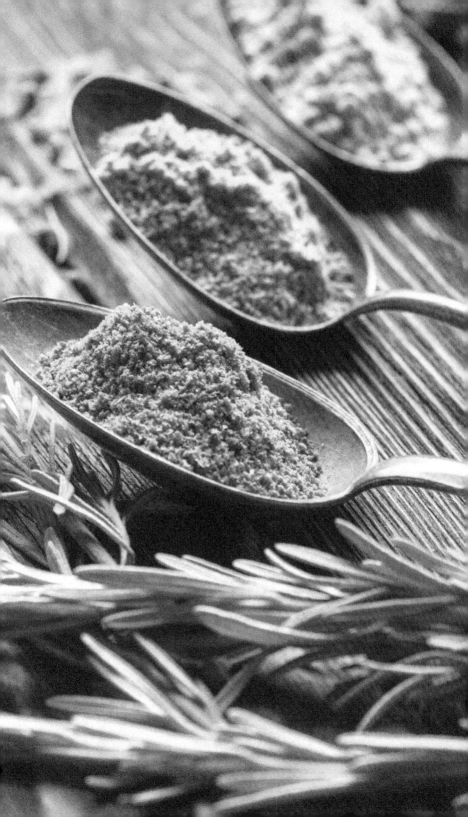

CHAPTER 9
APOTHECARY

therapeutic properties that offer natural remedies for a multitude of ailments. Each leaf and petal embodies a legacy of holistic healing and sensory delight, making herbal plants a timeless treasure in both gardens and households. The plants highlighted in this book are shown on the following pages and are just a small selection of those available to heal body and mind without pharmaceuticals.

Aloe Vera

Latin Name

Description ick, fleshy

leaves that

Medicinal and healing

properties, particularly for burns and skin

conditions.

Preferred Solvent: Water, glycerin

Arnica

Latin Name

Description ght yellow,

daisy-like fl

Medicinal uises, sprains,

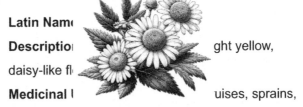

muscle soreness, and inflammation.

Preferred Solvent: Alcohol, oil

Ashwagandha

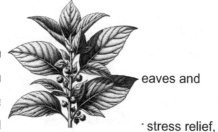

Latin Name

Description eaves and
yellow flowe

Medicinal · stress relief,
improving energy, and enhancing overall health.

Preferred Solvent: Alcohol, water

Basil

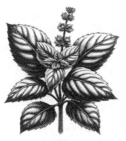

Latin Name

Description ad, green
leaves and

Medicinal ssues,
anti-inflammatory, and antibacterial properties.

Preferred Solvent: Alcohol, oil

Black Cohosh

Latin Name

Description 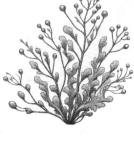 mpound
leaves and   es.
Medicinal   al symptoms
and PMS.

Preferred Solvent: Alcohol, water

Bladderwrack

Latin Name

Description   ir bladders
for buoyanc
Medicinal   lth and
weight loss.

Preferred Solvent: Alcohol, water

Calendula

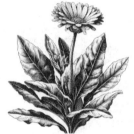

    Latin Name

    Description ꞁ flowers;
daisy-like a

    Medicinal ꞁ g,
anti-inflammatory, and antiseptic properties.

    Preferred Solvent: Oil, alcohol

Chamomile

    Latin Name

    Description h yellow
centers; fea

    Medicinal ꞁ gestive aid,
and anti-inflammatory properties.

    Preferred Solvent: Water, alcohol

Chaste Tree Berry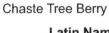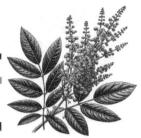

Latin Name

Description ⋯-like leaves
and purple

Medicinal ⋯balance, PMS,
and menopause symptoms.

Preferred Solvent: Alcohol, water

Chicory

Latin Name

Description ⋯ flowers;
dandelion-li

Medicinal ⋯ealth and liver
detoxification.

Preferred Solvent: Water, alcohol

Chlorella

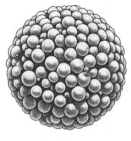

    Latin Nam

    Descriptio ɪae.

    Medicinal ɪ on, immune

    support, an ɪn.

    Preferred Solvent: Water

Comfrey

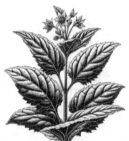

    Latin Nam

    Descriptio d bell-shaped

    flowers (puɪ

    Medicinal ɪ ɪling, bone

repair, and anti-inflammatory properties.

    Preferred Solvent: Oil, alcohol

Damiana

    Latin Name

    Description   atic, serrated
leaves and

    Medicinal   c properties,
mood enhancement, and digestive aid.

    Preferred Solvent: Alcohol, water

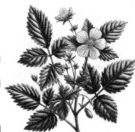

Dandelion

    Latin Name

    Description   nd toothed
leaves; milk

    Medicinal   diuretic, and
digestive health.

    Preferred Solvent: Water, alcohol

Dong Quai

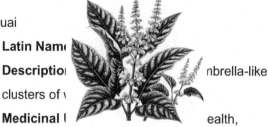

Latin Name

Description nbrella-like
clusters of

Medicinal ealth,

particularly menstrual and menopausal issues.

Preferred Solvent: Alcohol, water

Echinacea

Latin Name

Description large,
daisy-like fl disk.

Medicinal mune system
and reduce inflammation.

Preferred Solvent: Alcohol, water

Elderberry

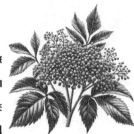

    Latin Name

    Description leaves and
clusters of s

    Medicinal ipport and
respiratory health.

    Preferred Solvent: Water, alcohol

Elderflower

    Latin Name

    Description small, white
flowers.

    Medicinal health,
anti-inflammatory, and diuretic properties.

    Preferred Solvent: Water, alcohol

Eucalyptus

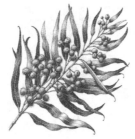

Latin Name

Description n leaves and
white, fluffy

Medicinal health,
antimicrobial properties, and pain relief.

Preferred Solvent: Oil, alcohol

Fennel

Latin Name

Description ellow
umbrella-sh

Medicinal ealth, anti-
inflammatory, and lactation support.

Preferred Solvent: Water, alcohol

Garlic

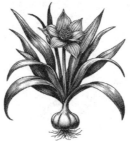

Latin Name

Description ery skin and
segmented

Medicinal ular health,
antimicrobial, and immune support.

Preferred Solvent: Oil, water

Ginger

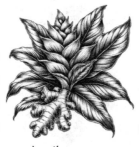

Latin Name

Description with a
pungent arc

Medicinal ssues, anti-
inflammatory, and anti-nausea properties.

Preferred Solvent: Alcohol, water

Ginkgo Biloba

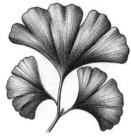

> **Latin Name**
>
> **Description** ...ped leaves.
>
> **Medicinal** ...upport,
>
> memory en...on.
>
> **Preferred Solvent**: Alcohol, water

Goldenseal

> **Latin Name**
>
> **Description** ...inkled, green
>
> leaves and
>
> **Medicinal** ...al properties,
>
> digestive health, and immune support.
>
> **Preferred Solvent**: Alcohol, water

Gotu Kola

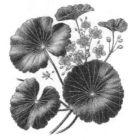

Latin Name

Description leaves with a
trailing grov

Medicinal upport, wound
healing, and skin health.

Preferred Solvent: Alcohol, water

Hibiscus

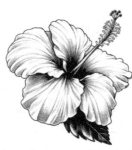

Latin Name

Description ful flowers
(commonly

Medicinal ular health,
digestive aid, and as an antioxidant.

Preferred Solvent: Water

Holy Basil

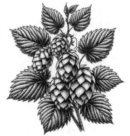

Latin Name

Description en or purple leaves and

Medicinal f, immune support, and anti-inflammatory properties.

Preferred Solvent: Alcohol, water

Hops

Latin Name

Description e-like flowers.

Medicinal ort, anxiety relief, and c

Preferred Solvent: Alcohol, water

Horseradish

Latin Name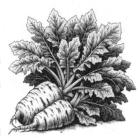

Description ge, rough
leaves and e root.

Medicinal health,
digestive aid, and antimicrobial properties.

Preferred Solvent: Water, alcohol

Horsetail

Latin Name

Description , hollow,
jointed sten ail.

Medicinal properties,
bone health, and skin conditions.

Preferred Solvent: Alcohol, water

Lavender

Latin Name

Description ...nder, gray-green ... spikes.

Medicinal ... eep support, and skin care.

Preferred Solvent: Oil, alcohol

Lemon Balm

Latin Name

Description ...rated, heart-shaped lea... ...rs.

Medicinal ... gestive health, and antiviral properties.

Preferred Solvent: Alcohol, water

Licorice

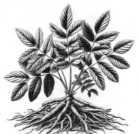

Latin Name

Description ᴵate leaves and small p

Medicinal ᴵ ealth, respiratory and anti-inflammatory suport.

Preferred Solvent: Alcohol, water

Maca

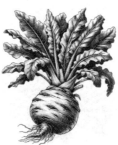

Latin Name

Description radish-like appearance

Medicinal ᴵ rmonal balance, and libido enhancement.

Preferred Solvent: Alcohol, water

Milk Thistle

Latin Name

Description flowers and
white-veine

Medicinal rt and
detoxification.

Preferred Solvent: Alcohol, water

Mint

Latin Name

Description rated leaves
and small p ers.

Medicinal ealth,
respiratory and anti-inflammatory support.

Preferred Solvent: Alcohol, water

Mullein

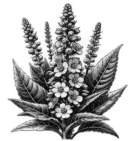

Latin Name

Description arge, wooly
leaves and

Medicinal health and
soothing irritated mucous membranes.

Preferred Solvent: Water, alcohol

Nettle

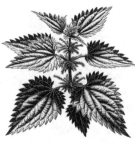

Latin Name

Description leaves and
small, gree s.

Medicinal matory,
diuretic, and allergy support.

Preferred Solvent: Alcohol, water

Oregano

Latin Name

Description il, green leaves and vers.

Medicinal al, digestive, and respiratory support.

Preferred Solvent: Alcohol, oil

Passionflower

Latin Name

Description cate flowers and lobed l

Medicinal ef, sleep support, and calming.

Preferred Solvent: Alcohol, water

Peppermint

    Latin Name

    Description k green,

    serrated lea vers.

    Medicinal ealth,

respiratory support, and pain relief.

    Preferred Solvent: Alcohol, water

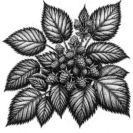

Raspberry

    Latin Name

    Description ns, pinnate

    leaves, and

    Medicinal ealth,

particularly during pregnancy and menstruation.

    Preferred Solvent: Water, alcohol

Red Clover

Latin Name

Description oliate leaves
and pink or

Medicinal)alance,

menopause symptoms, and skin health.

Preferred Solvent: Alcohol, water

Rhodiola

Latin Name

Description shy leaves
and yellow,

Medicinal f, cognitive

support, and energy enhancement.

Preferred Solvent: Alcohol, water

Rose

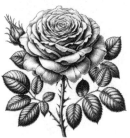

Latin Name

Description ny stems and
fragrant flo

Medicinal nood
enhancement, and anti-inflammatory properties.

Preferred Solvent: Water, oil

Rosemary

Latin Name

Description dle-like
leaves and

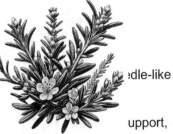

Medicinal upport,
digestive health, and antimicrobial properties.

Preferred Solvent: Alcohol, oil

Saffron

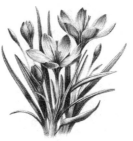

Latin Nam

Descriptio   ırple flowers
and red stiç

Medicinal l   ıncement,
digestive health, and antioxidant properties.

Preferred Solvent: Alcohol, water

Sage

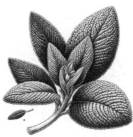

Latin Nam

Descriptio   y-green
leaves and

Medicinal l   upport, anti-
inflammatory, and antimicrobial properties.

Preferred Solvent: Alcohol, oil

Shatavari

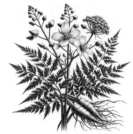

Latin Name

Description edle-like
leaves and

Medicinal ealth,
particularly hormonal balance and reproductive
support.

Preferred Solvent: Alcohol, water

Spirulina

Latin Name

Description a spiral shape.

Medicinal rient content,
immune su perties.

Preferred Solvent: Water

St. John's Wort

> **Latin Name**
>
> **Description** 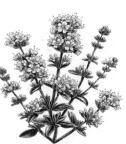 llow flowers
>
> and perfora
>
> **Medicinal** ancement,
>
> particularly for mild to moderate depression.
>
> **Preferred Solvent**: Alcohol, oil

Thyme

> **Latin Name**
>
> **Description** all, grey-green
>
> leaves and
>
> **Medicinal** health,
>
> antimicrobial properties, and digestive aid.
>
> **Preferred Solvent**: Alcohol, oil

Tribulus

Latin Name

Description with yellow
flowers and

Medicinal ncement and
muscle strength.

Preferred Solvent: Alcohol, water

Turmeric

Latin Name

Description large leaves
and yellow-

Medicinal matory,
antioxidant, and digestive health.

Preferred Solvent: Alcohol, oil

Valerian

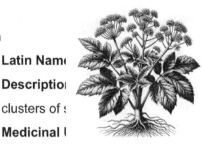

Latin Name

Description eaves and clusters of rs.

Medicinal ort and anxiety relief.

Preferred Solvent: Alcohol, water

Yarrow

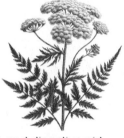

Latin Name

Description thery leaves and clusters owers.

Medicinal ling, anti-inflammatory, and digestive aid.

Preferred Solvent: Alcohol, water

Ylang-Ylang

Latin Name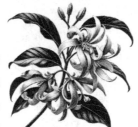

Description ⊃ing, fragrant

yellow flow

Medicinal ɪncement,

relaxation, and skin health.

Preferred Solvent: Oil, alcohol

I hope that the passion and the knowledge that I have shared has inspired you to begin your journey into the realm of herbal medicine and has served to demystify the terminology and techniques involved in the holistic management of your health. I also hope that you will see

AFTERWORD

that the integration of herbal remedies into your daily routine can be easily achieved without great adjustment.

Many women, who seek agency over their lives and health, can be discouraged by what may seem to be the impenetrable world of herbalism or may be skeptical of its effectiveness - I have shown however, that the gifts given to us by the natural world and their efficacy is backed by science and can be a very effective supplement to modern medicine.

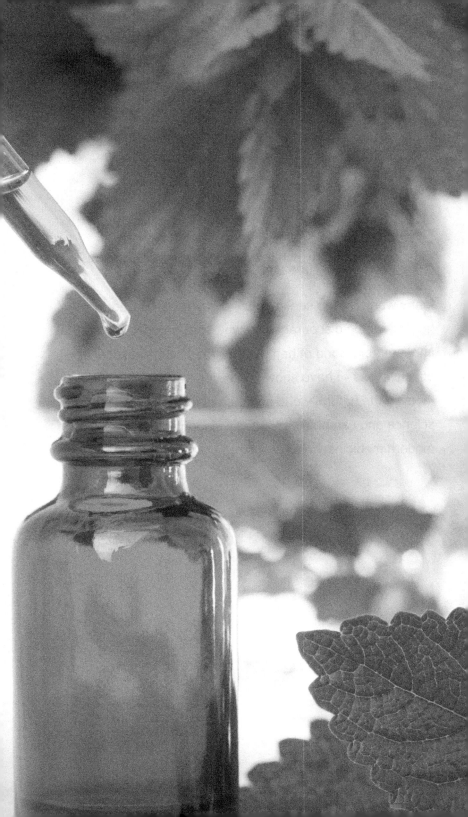

REFERENCES

otepotiintegrativehealth.co.nz/post/10-herbs-for-female-hor-mone-balance

- **Storing Dried Herbs and Herbal Preparations for Freshness** ... *https://chestnutherbs.com/storing-dried-herbs-and-herbal-preparations/*
- **Herbal tinctures: 6 types and recipes - MedicalNews Today** *https://www.medicalnewstoday.com/articles/324149*
- **How to Create Your Own Herbal Tea Blends** *https://blog.mountainroseherbs.com/guide-tea-blending*
- **A Beginner's Guide to Making Herbal Salves and Lotions** *https://www.healthline.com/health/diy-herbal-salves*
- **Poultice: How to Make an Herbal, Epsom Salt or Onion Type** *https://draxe.com/beauty/poultice/*
- **A preliminary review of studies on adaptogens** *https://www.ncbi.nlm.nih.gov/pmc/articles/PMC6240259/*
- **Dietary supplements and herbal remedies for pre-menstrual** ... *https://www.ncbi.nlm.nih.gov/books/NBK72353/*

- **Female infertility and herbal medicine: An over-view of the** ... *https://www.ncbi.nlm.nih.gov/pmc/articles/PMC8498057/*
- **The Effect of Salvia Officinalis on Hot Flashes in** ... **- NCBI** *https://www.ncbi.nlm.nih.gov/pmc/articles/PMC10363264/*
- **Effects of lavender on anxiety: A systematic review**

and meta ... *https://www.sciencedirect.com/science/article/pii/S0944711319303411#:~:text=The%20quantitative%20synthesis%20showed%20that,mean%20difference%20%3D%20%E2%88%925.99%20%5B95*

- **Valerian Root Dosage for Anxiety and Sleep** *https://www.healthline.com/health/food-nutrition/valerian-root*
- **St. John's Wort and Depression: In Depth | NCCIH** *https://www.nccih.nih.gov/health/st-johns-wort-and-depression-in-depth*
- **A Systematic Review and Meta-Analysis of Ginkgo biloba ...** *https://www.ncbi.nlm.nih.gov/pmc/articles/PMC3679686/*
- **12 Science-Backed Benefits of Peppermint Tea and Extracts** *https://www.healthline.com/nutrition/peppermint-tea*
- **Milk Thistle: Effects on Liver Disease and Cirrhosis ...** *https://www.ncbi.nlm.nih.gov/books/NBK11896/*
- **Prebiotic Potential of Herbal Medicines Used in Digestive ...** *https://www.ncbi.nlm.nih.gov/pmc/articles/PMC6065514/*
- **Antiinflammatory effects of turmeric (Curcuma longa) and ...** *https://www.sciencedirect.com/science/article/pii/B9780128192184000110*
- **Simplifying Herbal Skin Care: 5 Basic Recipes To Get You Started** *https://theherbalacademy.com/blog/5-basic-herbal-skin-care-recipes/*
- **Role and Mechanisms of Phytochemicals in Hair Growth ...** *https://www.ncbi.nlm.nih.gov/pmc/articles/PMC9963650/*
- **Herbal Treatment for Dermatologic Disorders** *https://www.ncbi.nlm.nih.gov/books/NBK92761/*
- **Herbal cosmetics in ancient India - PMC** *https://www.ncbi.nlm.nih.gov/pmc/articles/PMC2825132/*

- **Elderberry Supplementation Reduces Cold Duration and** ... *https://www.ncbi.nlm.nih.gov/pmc/articles/PMC4848651/*
- **What are Adaptogens & Types** *https://my.clevelandclinic.org/health/drugs/22361-adaptogens*
- *Herbal medicines for treatment of bacterial infections: a review* ... *https://academic.oup.com/jac/article/51/2/241/748873*
alance your Hormones *https://www.healthline.com/nutrition/herbs-that-balance-hormones*
- **Growing Medicinal Herbs in Pots: 10 Healing Plants** ... *https://chestnutherbs.com/growing-medicinal-herbs-in-pots/*
- **How to Make Herbal Salves https://blog.mountainroseherbs.com/diy-herbal-salves**
- **The Benefits of Fermented Herbs** *https://livingalchemy.com/blogs/blog/the-benefits-of-fermented-herbs*
- **Herbal Medicine Today: Clinical and Research Issues - PMC** *https://www.ncbi.nlm.nih.gov/pmc/articles/PMC2206236/*
- **Johns Hopkins Medicine. (n.d.). Anatomy of the endocrine system. Johns Hopkins Medicine.** *https://www.hopkinsmedicine.org/health/wellness-and-prevention/anatomy-of-the-endocrine-system*
- **Mount Sinai. (n.d.). Milk thistle. Mount Sinai Health Library** *https://www.mountsinai.org/health-library/herb/milk-thistle#:~:text=Silymarin%20has%20antioxidant%20and%20anti,in%20human%20studies%20are%20mixed*
- **Breast Cancer Prevention Partners. (n.d.). Phytoestrogens. BCPP** *https://www.bcpp.org/resource/phytoestrogens/#:~:text=Phytoestrogens%20are%20plant%20nutrients%20found,decreased%20risk%20of%20breast%20cancer*
- **Huzar, T. (2019, November 2). What to know about**

somatization. Medical News Today *https://www.medicalnew-stoday.com/articles/326847*

- **WebMD. (n.d.). Inulin: Uses, side effects, interactions, dosage, and warning** *https://www.webmd.com/vitamins/ai/ingredientmono-1048/inulin*

- **Cleveland Clinic. (n.d.). Cytokines. Cleveland Clinic** *https://my.clevelandclinic.org/health/body/24585-cytokines*

- **ScienceDirect. (n.d.). Catechin. ScienceDirect.** *https://www.sciencedirect.com/topics/agricultural-and-biological-sciences/catechin#:~:text=Catechins%20are%20a%20major%20group,their%20biological%20activities%20%5B74%5D*

- **WebMD. (n.d.). Phytonutrients: What you should know** *https://www.webmd.com/diet/phytonutrients-faq*

- **News-Medical. (n.d.). What is Somatization?** **News-Medical** *https://www.news-medical.net/health/What-is-Somatization.aspx#:~:text=Somatization%20is%20the%20expression%20of,back%20pain%2C%20nausea%20or%20fatigue.*

- **Mount Sinai. (n.d.). Rosemary** *https://www.mountsinai.org/health-library/herb/rosemary#:~:text=Because%20higher%20doses%20of%20rosemary,colitis%20should%20not%20take%20rosemary.*

Made in United States
Orlando, FL
28 December 2024